TIME AND PERFORMER TRAINING

Time and Performer Training addresses the importance and centrality of time and temporality to the practices, processes and conceptual thinking of performer training. Notions of time are embedded in almost every aspect of performer training, and so contributors to this book look at:

- age/aging and children in the training context
- how training impacts over a lifetime
- the duration of training and the impact of training regimes over time
- concepts of timing and the 'right' time
- how time is viewed from a range of international training perspectives
- collectives, ensembles and fashions in training, their decay or endurance.

Through focusing on time and the temporal in performer training, this book offers innovative ways of integrating research into studio practices. It also steps out beyond the more traditional places of training to open up time in relation to contested training practices that take place online, in festival spaces and in folk or amateur practices.

Ideal for both instructors and students, each section of this well–illustrated book follows a thematic structure and includes full–length chapters alongside shorter provocations. Featuring contributions from an international range of authors who draw on their backgrounds as artists, scholars and teachers, *Time and Performer Training* is a major step in our understanding of how time affects the preparation for performance.

Mark Evans is Professor of Theatre Training at Coventry University. He trained with Jacques Lecoq in Paris and has published widely on performer training and physical theatre, including: *Movement Training for the Modern Actor* (2009), *The Routledge Companion to Jacques Lecoq* (2016) and *Performance, Movement and the Body* (2019).

Konstantinos Thomaidis is Lecturer in Drama, Theatre & Performance at the University of Exeter and the Artistic Director of AdriftPM. He is founding co-editor of the *Journal of Interdisciplinary Voice Studies* and the *Routledge Voice Studies* series. His latest book is *Theatre & Voice* (2017).

Libby Worth is Reader in Contemporary Performance at Royal Holloway. She trained with Anna Halprin and in the Feldenkrais Method. She is co-editor of the journal *Theatre, Dance and Performance Training* and her most recent book is *Jasmin Vardimon's Dance Theatre: Movement, Memory and Metaphor* (2017).

TIME AND PERFORMER TRAINING

Edited by Mark Evans, Konstantinos Thomaidis and Libby Worth

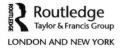
Routledge
Taylor & Francis Group

LONDON AND NEW YORK

First published 2019
by Routledge
2 Park Square, Milton Park, Abingdon, Oxon OX14 4RN

and by Routledge
52 Vanderbilt Avenue, New York, NY 10017

Routledge is an imprint of the Taylor & Francis Group, an informa business

British Library Cataloguing-in-Publication Data
A catalogue record for this book is available from the British Library

Library of Congress Cataloging-in-Publication Data
Names: Evans, Mark, 1957– editor. |
Thomaidis, Konstantinos, editor. | Worth, Libby, 1955– editor.
Title: Time and performer training / edited by Mark Evans,
Konstantinos Thomaidis and Libby Worth.
Description: Abingdon, Oxon; New York, NY: Routledge, 2019. |
Includes bibliographical references and index.
Identifiers: LCCN 2018048261 | ISBN 9780815396277 (hardback: alk. paper) |
ISBN 9780815396284 (paperback: alk. paper) | ISBN 9781351180368 (ebook) |
ISBN 9781351180351 (Adobe Reader) | ISBN 9781351180344 (ePub3) |
ISBN 9781351180337 (mobipocket unencrypted)
Subjects: LCSH: Acting. | Actors—Training of. | Space and time in the theater.
Classification: LCC PN2061 .T56 2019 | DDC 792.02/8—dc23
LC record available at https://lccn.loc.gov/2018048261

ISBN: 978-0-8153-9627-7 (hbk)
ISBN: 978-0-8153-9628-4 (pbk)
ISBN: 978-1-351-18036-8 (ebk)

Typeset in Bembo
by codeMantra

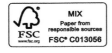

To Chronos and Kairos

CONTENTS

FIGURES

TABLES

CONTRIBUTORS

Anne Bogart is a Co-Artistic Director of the ensemble-based SITI Company, Head of the MFA Directing program at Columbia University and author of five books: *A Director Prepares*, *The Viewpoints Book*, *And Then You Act*, *Conversations with Anne* and *What's the Story*. With SITI, Bogart has directed more than 30 works in venues around the world, including *The Bacchae*, *Chess Match #5*, *Steel Hammer*, *The Theater is a Blank Page*, *Persians*, *A Rite*, *Café Variations,* *Radio Macbeth*, *American Document*, *bobrauschenbergamerica* and *Hotel Cassiopeia*. Recent opera works include Handel's *Alcina*, Dvorak's *Dimitrij*, Verdi's *Macbeth*, Bellini's *Norma* and Bizet's *Carmen*. Her many awards and fellowships include three honorary doctorates (Cornish School of the Arts, Bard College and Skidmore College), a Duke Artist Fellowship, a United States Artists Fellowship, a Guggenheim Fellowship, a Rockefeller/Bellagio Fellowship and a Robert Rauschenberg Foundation Residency Fellowship.

Patrick Campbell is a theatre practitioner and academic, and Senior Lecturer in Drama at Manchester Metropolitan University (UK). His research is both theoretical and practice-based, and focuses on the ways in which artists working within a postdramatic theatrical paradigm in Europe and Latin America are challenging monolithic, phallogocentric framings of subjectivity, representability and heritage through performance and training. As an artist, Patrick has directed and performed in site-specific and immersive theatre performances that explore the liminal space between myth, biography and autobiography, working in close collaboration with companies and institutions, such as the Contact Theatre Manchester (UK), Triangle Theatre (UK), COSmino Theatre (Germany) and the Teatro Vila Velha (Brazil).

Kate Craddock is a Senior Lecturer at Northumbria University, Newcastle where she is Programme Leader on the industry-focused MA Theatre and Performance programme. Kate is also Founder and Festival Director of GIFT: Gateshead International Festival of Theatre, an annual artist-led festival celebrating contemporary theatre. As a theatre-maker, Kate has presented her own performance work at venues and festivals across the UK and internationally. Kate is on the Board of Trustees for the award winning Paper Birds Theatre Company and for ARC Stockton Arts Centre. Kate is a 2018/19 Clore Fellow with The Clore Leadership Programme.

Mark Evans is an Associate Dean and Professor of Theatre Training and Education in the Faculty of Arts and Humanities at Coventry University. He trained at the École Jacques Lecoq, in Paris. He is an Associate Editor of the *Theatre Dance and Performance Training* journal and has published widely on performer training and physical theatre, including *Jacques Copeau* (2006, 2nd ed. 2018), *Movement Training for the Modern Actor* (2009), *The Actor Training Reader* (2013) and *The Routledge Companion to Jacques Lecoq* (2016). His latest book, *Performance, Movement and the Body*, will be published by Palgrave in February 2019.

Mark Hamilton is a Senior Lecturer (World Stages) at Regent's University London. He first studied at the University of Birmingham, where Nadine George educated him in her embodied voice practice. Extramurally, he explored Jerzy Grotowski's methodologies. Mark later trained in *bharatanatyam, astanga vinyasa yoga* and *kalaripayattu*. For thirteen years, he was close collaborator of Mika, seminal queer Maori artist. Mark's doctoral thesis awarded by the University of Canterbury (NZ) explored the interface of the martial arts and dance. Mark's research explores intercultural performance. He explores the interface of European experimental theatre, performance ethnography and queer live art.

Jennifer Jackson's career spans performing, choreographing, writing and teaching. A former soloist with the Royal Ballet, she danced principal roles in the major classics and new works by Ashton and MacMillan. Her choreography includes commissioned work for ballet companies, fringe theatre, research projects and vocational students. Prior to joining London Studio Centre in 2015 as Artistic Director of Images Ballet Company, she was Senior Lecturer in Dance Studies at University of Surrey and choreography tutor at the Royal Ballet School for 16 years. Her writing is published in professional and academic journals including *Dancing Times* and *Research in Dance Education*.

Tim Jones specialized over the last 35 years in intercultural research and performance, with particular interest in voice and sound and with outcomes across different forms (music, theatre, storytelling) and media (theatre, T.V., film). From 1984, as a member of Pan Project to recent collaborations with *gender wayang* ensemble Segara Madu, Tim's performance, community projects and teaching have focused on accessibility for all. Current practice includes: development of 'Songworlds' for therapeutic use; 'Hesitant Human Being' – adventures in reconciliation, a lecture/performance piece; ongoing Group Relations Conference *Energy, Creative Collaboration and Wellbeing* for Il Nodo Group, Italy. Tim is an Amerta Movement Practitioner and teacher. www.thenatureofsound.com

Chan E. Park is the author of *Voices from the Straw Mat: Toward an Ethnography of Korean Story Singing* (University of Hawai'i Press 2003), and currently Professor of Korean Literature and Performance at Ohio State University. Park has innovated numerous bilingual and theatrical *pansori* including: *In 1903, Pak Hungbo Went to Hawai'i* (2003); *When Tiger Smoked His Pipe* (2003); *Shim Chong: A Korean Folktale* (2003); *Alaskan Pansori: Klanott and the Land Otter People* (2005); *Song of Everyday Chunhyang* (2008); and *Hare Returns from the Underwater Palace* (2013).

Eugénie Pastor is an artist, performer and musician. She is a member of award-winning Little Bulb Theatre, with whom she co-devised and performed *Operation Greenfield* (2010), *Orpheus* (2013) and *The Future* (2019), among others. She founded She Goat with fellow Little Bulb artist Shamira Turner. Their debut show *DoppelDänger* (2017), performed by a pair of real-life doppelgängers, explores the boundaries between theatre and live music and what it means to be two women on stage. As an independent artist, Eugénie created *Pube* (2016), a one-on-one piece exploring our relationship with pubic hair. Eugénie has a Ph.D. in Drama and Theatre Studies from Royal Holloway, University of London, and she is a part-time lecturer in Drama and Performance at London South Bank University.

Diego Pellecchia is an Associate Professor in the Faculty of Cultural Studies of Kyoto Sangyō University. He received his Ph.D. in Drama and Theatre Studies at Royal Holloway, University of London with a thesis on the reception of Japanese Noh theatre in the West. His numerous research projects include amateur Noh practice, Noh and digital humanities, Noh and memory. He studies and performs Noh under the guidance of Master-Actor Udaka Michishige (Kongō School). In 2013, he performed his first complete Noh as protagonist.

Jonathan Pitches is a Professor of Theatre and Performance at the University of Leeds and specializes in the study of performer training, environmental performance and blended learning. He is founding co-editor of the journal of *Theatre, Dance and Performance Training* and has published several books in this area including *Vsevolod Meyerhold* (2003/18), *Science and the Stanislavsky Tradition of Acting* (2006/9) *Russians in Britain* (2012) and *Stanislavsky in the World* (with Dr Stefan Aquilina 2017). He is editor of *Great Stage Directors Vol 3: Komisarjevsky, Copeau, Guthrie* (2018) and sole author of *Performing Mountains* (forthcoming 2019), supported by the AHRC.

Gyllian Raby is an Associate Professor at Brock University's Department of Dramatic Arts in Ontario, Canada. She was the founding artistic director of One Yellow Rabbit Performance Theatre, chronicled in Martin Morrow's book *Wild Theatre*, and also led Northern Light Theatre, working across Canada and in the US. In 2018, her adaptation of Nicolai Erdman's *The Suicide* was staged by the Cork School of Music; her project *We Who Know Nothing About Hiawatha Are Proud to Present Hiawatha* was played in the Soil Festival and her production of *Sabina's Splendid Brain* with Stolen Theatre opened the Luce Irigaray Philosophy Circle.

Adriana La Selva is a Brazilian theatre-maker based in Belgium where she works as freelance artist and teacher. She is currently a Ph.D. candidate at the University of Ghent in Belgium and School of Arts Ghent (KASK) in collaboration with the a.pass Institute (Brussels), investigating contemporary performer training processes and politics of embodied research.

Evi Stamatiou is a Senior Lecturer in Theatre at the University of Chichester, UK. Her research interests include performer training, socially engaged theatre, musical theatre and practice as research. Evi is a Ph.D. candidate at the Royal Central School of Speech and Drama, University of London. She is an award-winning actor, writer and director who works across stage and screen. She has presented her work in Greece, United Kingdom, Germany, Poland, Estonia, South Africa, Brazil, France and the United States. She has published essays with various academic publishers including Routledge, Intellect Books, Palgrave MacMillan, MacFarland & Co and Bloomsbury/Methuen Drama.

Tiffany Strawson lived in Bali from 1998 to 2012 and pursued a mask training which involved studying the carving, dance and embodiment of the Balinese *topeng* mask and its application in a traditional context. Tiffany continues to learn the ceremonial practices associated with *topeng* performances those being the philosophical principles underlying the choreography, stories and mantras. Previously, Tiffany artistically produced the Bali-Unmasked Project which promotes intercultural exchange to and from Bali and now works as a performance-maker and cultural commissioner of intercultural, devised theatre. Tiffany has published in *TDPT* and *Asian Theatre Journal*.

Jenny Swingler trained at the École Jacques Lecoq (2008–2011) as part of the Acting program and at the school's Laboratory of Movement Study under the architect Krikor Belekian. In 2018, she was awarded a TECHNE scholarship and is currently embarking on a practice-based Ph.D. in *Performing Imagined Geographies* at the University of Roehampton. As Co-Artistic Director of Clout Theatre she has taken work to The Roundhouse, Battersea Arts Centre, Meyerhold Theatre Centre, Istanbul City Theatre and the Beijing People's Art Theatre.

Udaka Tatsushige was born in Kyoto in 1981. He trained under the 26th head of the Kongō school, Kongō Hisanori, and his father, Udaka Michishige. He took his first role as *kokata* (child actor) when he was three years old. Besides his career on stage, he teaches noh chant and dance, and is actively involved in the dissemination of noh to younger audiences through workshops and lectures. He performed in Japan, as well as also in South Korea, France, Germany, Great Britain and in the U.S. In 2015, he inaugurated his performance series, the *Tatsushige no Kai*.

Konstantinos Thomaidis is Lecturer in Drama, Theatre & Performance at the University of Exeter. He is founding co-editor of the *Routledge Voice Studies* book series and the *Journal of Interdisciplinary Voice Studies* and founding co-convener of the 'Sound, Voice & Music' working group at TaPRA. He co-edited *Voice Studies: Critical Approaches to Process, Performance and Experience* (Routledge 2015) and the special issue 'Voicing Belonging: Traditional Singing in a Globalized World' (Intellect 2017), and wrote *Theatre & Voice* (Palgrave/Springer 2017). He is currently editing the special issue 'What Is New in Voice Training?' for the *Theatre, Dance and Performance Training* journal. He is the Artistic Director of Adrift Performance Makers.

Darren Tunstall has been an actor, director and writer since 1988, including for the Royal Shakespeare Company, the National Theatre, BBC, ITV, Film Four and as part of the 'physical theatre' movement during the 1990s. Since 2015, he has been a lecturer at the Guildford School of Acting, University of Surrey. He has written for *The Routledge Companion to Theatre, Performance and Cognitive Science, The Routledge Companion to Actors' Shakespeare, The Routledge Companion to Jacques Lecoq, Shakespeare Bulletin* and *Journal of Adaptation in Film and Performance*. His book *Shakespeare and Gesture in Practice* was published in 2016.

Jane Turner is the author of the Routledge Performance Practitioners book *Eugenio Barba* (2004, 2nd edition 2018); she has also published material on Third Theatre, Balinese theatre, performer training, theatre ethnography, the sublime and contemporary theatre performances. She is currently embarked on research into the training, dramaturgy and participatory strategies employed by the Third Theatre community with Patrick Campbell, particularly in Latin America and Europe. As an academic at Manchester Metropolitan University, she teaches on the Contemporary Theatre and Performance degree.

Laura Vorwerg is a Ph.D. candidate at Royal Holloway, University of London, and is also currently engaged as a Visiting Lecturer. Her research focuses on interdisciplinary performance practice and seeks to examine the ways in which embodied physical skills are taught, learnt, maintained and adapted within professional practice. She has previously worked as a freelance director in opera and theatre.

David Wiles is Emeritus Professor of Drama at the University of Exeter, having spent much of his career at Royal Holloway, University of London. He is the author of *Theatre & Time* (Palgrave, 2016). His interest in 'time' grew out of research into space that culminated in *A Short History of Western Performance Space* (CUP, 2003). He has published extensively in the fields of Greek and Elizabethan theatre, and is currently working on a history of the rhetorical tradition of acting. He hopes that retirement will allow him time in the future to tackle a history of the acting process.

Libby Worth is a Reader in Contemporary Performance Practices in the Department of Drama, Theatre and Dance, Royal Holloway, University of London. She is a movement practitioner who specializes in site-responsive interdisciplinary performance and who trained in the Feldenkrais Method and in dance with Anna Halprin. She is co-editor of the *Theatre, Dance and Performer Training* journal. Published texts include *Anna Halprin* (2004, co-authored, 2nd ed. 2018), *Ninette de Valois: Adventurous Traditionalist* (2012, co-edited, 2nd ed. 2018), *Jasmin Vardimon's Dance Theatre: Movement, Memory and Metaphor* (2016) and chapters/articles on Mabel Todd, Jenny Kemp, Caryl Churchill, Robert Helpmann, the Feldenkrais Method and on Dance Improvisation.

ACKNOWLEDGEMENTS

The editors would like to thank all the contributors to the TaPRA Working Group on Performer Training at the TaPRA Annual Conference, 8–10 September 2015, University of Worcester. We would also like to thank Ben Piggott and Laura Soppelsa at Routledge for their support and guidance in the preparation of this book. The editors are grateful to their respective institutions, Coventry University, University of Exeter and Royal Holloway University of London, for support given to research projects such as this.

A special thanks goes to Natalia Theodoridou, Paul Brill and Vanessa Oakes for their love, support and patience.

SECTION I
(Re)Introducing time

1

FOREWORD

Embodied time

Anne Bogart

As a mid-year transfer student at Bard College, I stood on a long line to sign up for a popular theatre class taught by Bill Driver, the chair of the theatre department who would soon become my first directing teacher. Sitting quietly at a small desk, Driver seemed to ignore the frantic atmosphere of impatient students vying for places in his classes. After what felt like an interminable wait, I finally stood before him, surprised to find him relaxed and present with me, interested in who I was and where I came from. Despite the surrounding chaos, he seemed neither rushed nor hurried. He paid no attention to the roiling line of irritated students behind me. This demonstration of patience and his attitude of one-thing-at-a-time became my first lesson in directing from Bill Driver.

Human life spans a relatively short and unpredictable arc of time, and the nagging question of how to handle the day-to-day encounters and trials can be challenging. We are born worriers, and I am no exception. Without tempering my natural proclivity to hurry, I tend to rush around in order to make things happen. I try to fill the gaps with activity and distraction. I agonize constantly about how well I am doing in comparison to others, and I fret about what I am missing out on. But with vigilance and restraint in my relation to time, I can temper these tendencies.

My perception of time is generally subjective and alters in relation to my inner state, emotions and moods. For example, I make everyday decisions such as whether to take the elevator or the stairs based on an anticipation of duration linked to my current feeling about time passing. I notice that time seems to speed up when I am enjoying myself and then it slows down again during periods of what might be considered boredom. But the notion of boredom may be misleading. By being in the moment, attentive to the surroundings and to the people, I can allow the opportunity for a deeper penetration of time. Intervals of time feel longer when I pay close attention to the present moment and allow for the array of differentiated perceptions that are within my grasp.

In order not to be overwhelmed by the limitations of time, I endeavour to deliberately develop a constructive inner posture in relation to the present moment. I try to remember to consciously choose an attitude appropriate to the particular pressures inherent in any given situation. I try to be sensitive to the difference between horizontal and vertical times.

When busy, when trying to get from where I am to where I want to be, I am generally living in horizontal time. Horizontal time is linear and has a past that is remembered and a future that is imagined. Horizontal time can make me feel under pressure and slight and insignificant. Vertical time, in contrast, may contain horizontal time but it also intersects and disrupts the experience of linear time. Vertical time arrives in small doses and has no past and no future outside of the present moment. In vertical time, *nowness* is absolutely real and non-divisible. Experiencing vertical time, I am more awake. I feel more and see more. I notice the mist rising off a meadow. I taste each sip in a cup of fragrant afternoon tea. I can fully enjoy an aimless walk at sunset. It is in vertical time that the conditions are ripe to experience epiphany.

Art creates the experience of vertical time for the perceiver by plunging a stake or dropping an anchor into the endless flow of time, thereby creating a sense of eternity in the human body. A van Gogh landscape painting offers a taste of eternity by allowing us, in its proximity, to experience vertical time. Music theorist Jonathan Kramer describes vertical time in music as a 'single present stretched out into enormous duration, a potentially infinite "now" that nonetheless feels like an instant' (1988: 55). In the experience of a musical performance, it is possible to reach a place where there is no differentiation between past, present and future. The experience of vertical time resets and refreshes us.

The theatre too has the capacity to generate moments of eternity by creating the conditions for an audience's experience of vertical time. The theatre shares with music the languages of time via tempo, duration or rhythm but also traffics in the semantics of space, encompassing architecture, shape or spatial relationship. While speaking in both the languages of time and of space, how do we create the conditions for eternity? How do we develop the ability to embody vertical time, to stop, to put on the brakes and bring the audience with us into the present moment?

Largely due to the fact that the day-to-day speed of our contemporary culture is accelerating at an alarming rate, the theatre in particular has the urgent task to provide audiences with alternate time signatures. It is possible and also necessary for theatre-makers to embody vertical time in order to be able to generate moments that transcend the rush of time. A theatre-maker's most consistent obstacle is time. We are all generally under the pressure of deadlines and financial restraints as well as doubts and fears about our own capabilities. In order for the theatre to set up the circumstances for an audience to experience vertical time, theatre-makers themselves must consistently undergo training in embodied time.

One of the basic tools that an actor must develop is the ability to relax. Because it is most difficult to relax under stress, effective theatre training purposefully creates stressful circumstances in order for the actor to seek ways to relax under pressure. Paradoxically, the actor must train aggressively in order to learn how to relax under stressful conditions. Sensitivity to time increases when anxiety decreases.

Training should also offer tools that animate an actor's receptivity to what is happening in the present moment and the ability to differentiate one moment, one sensation and one time signature, from the next. Peter Brook pointed out that it is easy to be sensitive in the fingers and the face, but an actor needs to become sensitive throughout the body. Sensitivity requires flexibility and openness to stimuli, and this in turn begets precision in stage movement as well as definition and clarity.

To embody time, one must practise being rooted in the middle, in the moment, rather than striving blindly and nervously towards a goal. Being in the middle requires one to consciously shift mindset from winning to an interest in exploring one's own stuckness and experimenting with where one is rather than what one wants to attain. Training should develop strategic patience. In the moment when one's ancient flight-or-fight impulses arise, it is possible, through practice, to apply the brakes, resist rushing, think fast and slow down at the same time.

My friend, the Dutch actress Saskia Noordhoek Hegt, described a theatre workshop led by a Buddhist monk. At the start of each session, the participants were required to get onto their hands and knees, and scrub the floor of the studio with cold water until told that they could stop and proceed with the day's work. Quite irritated by the necessity to clean an already spotless floor, Saskia's impatience intensified over time. One day, towards the end of the course, the participants were left cleaning the floor for what felt like an inordinate amount of time. Saskia's impatience and frustration with what felt like a futile task escalated until suddenly, in the midst of brushing the floor on her hands and knees, her anxiety fell away and she found herself smack dab in the present moment. She finally understood that this practice was the point of the workshop. She had learned how to cultivate vertical time.

I cherish the moments in art where, after a dramatic build and a period of what feels like roiling, searching and struggle, the whole thing stops and I am, as spectator, listener or viewer, suspended mid-air in what feels like eternity. In these precious moments, I feel as though I am falling. Vertical time offers a sense of vastness from the inside and can indeed feel like falling – falling into the arms of emptiness. In that moment, I remember that between the past and the future there exists lots of space. Vertical time peels back the layers to reveal the essence of life in the present moment.

SITI Company recently turned 25 years old. Why have we lasted so long? Perhaps it is because together, via training and experience, we continue to study the art of embodied time. We have learned to be patient with one another and relax under stress. In creating work, we continue to learn strategic patience, to purposefully wait for the solution to reveal itself. Where patience may have once felt like lack of control, we have learned that it is a form of control over the tempo of an ongoing flow of life that otherwise controls us. Patience is power. Restraint is a tool. We continue to learn and study how to increase receptivity to what is happening in the present moment and how to differentiate one moment, one sensation and one time signature, from the next. Together we practise being in the middle of a moment, exploring our stuckness with great interest, rather than racing towards the endpoint.

On tour with SITI Company to Minneapolis several years ago, I searched for and found a Saturday morning yoga class. Upon arriving at the yoga studio, I noticed a crowd of people waiting to get into the class. Not only had the receptionist not shown up, but also the computer was broken and the teacher for the scheduled class was obliged to check people in as well as teach the class, which by then was meant to have begun. The line of people trying to get into the weekend class was long, and everyone was growing impatient. I stood in the line, and when I arrived at the desk where the yoga teacher sat at the broken computer, I said to her, 'You are practising your yoga right now, aren't you.' She nodded slowly in assent.

Reference

Kramer, J. (1988) *The Time of Music: New Meanings, New Temporalities, New Listening Strategies*, New York: Schirmer/Mosel Verlag.

2

INTRODUCTION

Expansive temporalities of performer training

Konstantinos Thomaidis, with Mark Evans and Libby Worth

Training practices in dance, music, theatre and performance disciplines operate across a dense intermix of timelines, timescales and timetables. During training, learning activities take up time and can also become important indicators of time passing. The training itself can have demarcated beginnings and end points; somewhere in between, exercises involving rhythm, counting, metre or timing unfold in time. These temporal unfoldings are not linear by default. Repetition, interruption, pauses and gaps, all produce a wide array of temporal experiences for both teachers and learners. Such corporal experiences are inflected by larger timescales of pedagogic lineages and performance traditions, socially and culturally significant understandings of time, and prevailing histories of performance practices and genres. These, in turn, sit alongside individual processes of aging in and through training, the narratives trainees develop for themselves during and after their years in training (sometimes even before), and the cross-generational exchange built into the very fabric of pedagogy. The interplay of micro- and macro-temporalities can further translate into an encounter between time zones in the synchronous or asynchronous transnational exchange facilitated by online platforms and international festivals. Time in training also accrues ideological value in the way it embraces or undercuts future-oriented notions of productivity, continuity and regularity, or divisions between work and leisure. Given the proliferating encounters between performer training and time, how can we unpack their significance in meaningful ways? What new knowledges can emerge through a closer examination of the temporal make-up of performance pedagogy? What can a book on training, broadly conceived, add to discussions of time and temporality? And how does such analysis speak to current concerns of performance theorists and makers?

Turning to time: performance studies and the temporal turn

'Theatre, like history, is an art of time. Even, we could say, *the* art of time. Time is the stuffing of the stage – it's what actors, directors, and designers manipulate together,' writes Rebecca Schneider in *Theatre & History* (2014: 7; original emphasis). Her assertion draws implicitly on the fact that performers are time-bound, finite, material beings, their work occurring in specified time conditions. Further, her reference to 'manipulation' bestows special temporal powers upon performers. Be they actors, dancers or musicians, performers are expected – and in fact are able – to orchestrate time towards designed or desired outcomes. Whether deploying rhythm, pace and timing or enmeshing their personal histories and time-marked bodies with fictional and scenic times, their work routinely dwells on handling, controlling, exploiting, manoeuvring or, even, engineering the temporal dimension of the theatrical experience. In this sense, performers not only become operative as such within time; they also prompt specific operations of time into being.

This relationship between performing and time comes with a particular set of complexities. Take, for instance, the way performers engender presence or now-ness: 'The actor's "now,"' continues Schneider, 'is not the audience's "now," even as these "now"'s and "then"'s meet and bleed, paradoxically, into a shared moment' (2014: 40). For Jerzy Limon, this temporal paradox or disjuncture underlying the performer's work is crucial for the very emergence of performance:

> theatre arises from the appearance of discrepant time structures: the performer as a live actor, living in the same time as the spectator, pretends that they are someone from the past (or, more rarely, from the future), but behaves as if the fictional figure were living now, in congruence with the biological time of the actor and the spectator. This duality is perhaps the most important feature of stage time.
>
> *(2014: 217)*

The time(s) of performers and spectators can be both aligned and divergent, and the embodied present of the performer is made porous through its coexistence with other epochs – historical or fictional – and time signatures.

Early-21st-century performance studies found fertile critical ground in interrogating postulations of performance as an art primarily emerging in the present. Much of this scholarship originated in dialogue with Peggy Phelan's well-rehearsed argument that 'performance's only life is in the present' as it 'leaves no visible trace afterward' (1993: 146, 149). In a line of argumentation that gives transience in performance an ontological status, the moment of performance is posited as unable to be seized, the bodies partaking in it forever fleeting and mutable; in Phelan's oft-quoted maxim, 'Performance marks the body itself as loss' (1993: 148). Hans-Thies Lehmann, in his study of postdramatic theatre, suggested a further disappearance: of time itself. Aristotelian dramaturgies aimed '*to prevent the appearance of time as time.* Time as such is meant to disappear, to be reduced to an unnoticeable condition of being of the action' (Lehmann 2006: 161; original emphasis). By contrast, Lehmann affirms, post-Brechtian and post-dramatic aesthetics deploy strategies such as the prolongation of duration or repetition to unhinge the present of performance from its conventional ties to scenic temporality. Philip Auslander, as a counterargument to Phelan and conventional understandings of performance as a live event, contended that liveness, as an attribute of performance almost fetishisticly linked to ephemerality and evanescence, was in fact produced by the advent of recordability and mediatization. Rejecting any prioritization of the live, he suggested that 'live performance has indeed been pried from its shell and that all performance modes, live or mediatized, are now equal; none is perceived as auratic or authentic' (Auslander 2008: 50). The indissolubility of the present of performance was further questioned by arguments such as those put forward by Marvin Carlson (2001), who theorized performance as always haunted by previous performances, materials, spaces and practices; Diana Taylor (2003: xvii), who argued that performance itself, beyond its immediate present, acts as 'a nonarchival system of transfer' of a repertoire of socially significant knowledges; and Rebecca Schneider (2011), for whom re-enactments are productive means towards rethinking the relation of performance to its past, a past never seen as fully bygone.[1]

This corpus of work problematized theatre as an art unequivocally linked to presence – or, at least, predestined to performing presence in a limited number of ways – therefore opening up the field to a broader consideration of time and performativity. Until recently, writing in performance studies lamented the dearth of publications in the area. David Wiles, for example, stated that 'there is a conspicuous lack of broad-based books on time as the core of theatrical performance' (2014: 68), and, in Maurya Wickstrom's words, 'although theatre as a medium is strikingly fluent in and fluid with temporality, we have not perhaps been as engaged with temporality in its own right as some other disciplines have been' (2016). While these observations are fair, the situation has been rapidly changing. Jerzy Limon (2010, 2014) has systematically worked towards proposing a taxonomy of the various iterations of time structures in the theatre, ranging from fictional, historical and scenic time to the biological time of the actors, the duration of the performance in real time and the structural time produced by the semiotic systems at play (for example, the rhythm of verse in poetic text or of musical phrasing in operatic performance). Matthew D. Wagner's monograph *Shakespeare, Theatre and Time* (2012) unpacked temporality from the perspective of early modern theatre-going and argued for the predominance of three modes of engaging time in the performance of Shakespeare's plays: dissonance (chaotic, non-continuous temporality), materiality (time as taking bodied or object forms) and thickness (collusions of past, present and future).

David Wiles, on the other hand, in *Theatre & Time*, explored time from two perspectives: the first is the macro-level, which he called 'rhythms of the Earth' (2014: 15), referencing the historic and contemporary connections of theatre to the passage of time, the rotation of the seasons, festival time and holidays. The second, the micro-level of the 'rhythms of the body' (2014: 30–43), focuses on the generation of principles and understandings of rhythmicity in bodily rhythms, such as the heartbeat, in ways that are also attuned to what appears as normal rhythm to the audience of each era. Stuart Grant, Jodie McNeilly and Maeva Veerapen's edited collection *Performance and Temporalisation* brought together an international network of philosophers, performance scholars and artists to contemplate the 'affective, inconsistent, living, multiple, relative, perceptual dimension of time' (2015: 7). Time, emphasized here as subjective, is explored in an array of practices, including responsive architecture, intimate immersive performance, dance, intermedial installation or religious conversion. Lastly, David Ian Rabey's *Theatre, Time and Temporality* (2016) interwove an interdisciplinary selection of theories of time with close readings of Anglophone plays, from Shakespeare to debbie tucker green, to unlock the political potential of representing time in alternative ways in theatre. For Rabey,

> tasks for theatre might encompass a demonstratively embodied retooling process, aiming to re-temporalize the temporal, demonstrate as provisional what is purportedly 'fixed,' emphasize the transience of the supposedly permanent, expose the intrinsic flaws of the systemic ideologies underpinning current power structures and manifest the surprising possibilities that are alternative to what is widely supposed to be, and promoted as, natural, just and inevitable.
>
> *(2016: 199–200)*

Such palpable increase in academic publications,[2] placed alongside the debates of the previous decade around presence, evidences that theatre and performance studies is now an active participant in the 'temporal turn,' the systematic probing and re-evaluation of time across various fields of study.[3] Major conferences and research gatherings have taken theatre time or the performativity of time as their key thematic concerns, including 'Time/Transcendence/Performance' (Monash University 2009), 'NOW THEN: Performance and Temporality' (PSi, Stanford University 2013), 'Matters of Time' (Cambridge 2013), 'Presenting the Theatrical Past' (IFTR, Stockholm University 2016) and 'Troubling Time: An Exploration of Temporality in the Arts' (Manchester University 2017). Similarly, in recent years, the specialist journal *Performance Research* has published a number of special issues on facets of the temporal experience of performance, such as *On Duration* (Scheer 2012), *On Time* (Jakovljevic and Mantoan 2014), *On Repetition* (Kartsaki and Schmidt 2015) and *On Children* (Senior and The Institute for the Art and Practice of Dissent at Home 2018), while various doctoral projects have rethought time in theatre and performance across early modern plays, devising, musical theatre, live art and contemporary performance (Cull 2009; Ellis 2013; Manninen 2014; Kelly 2015; Wakefield 2016). Far from offering an unquestioned or undisputed background to the theatrical experience, time is now moving to the epicentre of performance studies as an issue of fundamental significance.

Performer training and making time(s)

Despite such proliferative discourses, most of the above studies have principally focused on the temporal facets of the encounter between performers and spectators or within processes of performance-making and devising, therefore excluding performer training as a primary area of interest. Schneider's or Limon's opening remarks are in fact short comments extrapolated from longer works that are largely not preoccupied with performer pedagogy. Similarly, it may be true that the experiential qualities of time have been central to most performer-training systems and methodologies, from Stanislavski's tempo–rhythm and Laban's combination of time with space, weight and flow to Bogart and Overlie's approaches to tempo, duration, kinesthetic response and repetition. However, there is still a remarkable lack of writing directly bridging time studies and the temporal turn within the field of performer training. This edited collection contributes to filling this gap through acknowledging the extent to which notions of time are embedded in almost every aspect of movement/dance, speech/voice and actor training, while also inviting systematic critical interrogation of temporality as conceived, perceived and practised by artists, trainers and trainees. It is, then, the primary aim of *Time and Performer Training* to address the disjunction between the centrality of time and temporality to the practices and processes of performer training and the paucity of conceptual thinking and scholarly publications explicitly dedicated to this subject.

Much of the existing performance studies literature on the subject of time hinges on the distinction between external, quantifiable, objectifiable, chronological or horological *time* and *temporality* as the embodied, emergent, relative and phenomenologically perceived I-experience of time, with an argument often developed for the necessity of closer attentiveness to the latter.[4] Given the unavoidability (if not primacy) of the I-perspective in pedagogic settings and practices, *Time and Performer Training* resonates with this aim but, further, wishes to explore the tensions, interconnections and porosity between these categories. If training is taken as the process of cultivating and endisciplining performers' bodies (Zarrilli 1990; Evans 2009), closer attention to the intersections of time and pedagogy can shed light on the processes through which cultures of time (divisions of labour, designations of appropriate time for training, conventions, traditions and aesthetics of rhythm, tempo, duration and metre, ideologies of time) become embodied and personal and, vice versa, the ways in which phenomenal temporalities intervene in specific understandings and contexts of time. The scope of this collection is deliberately wide – methodologically, geographically, disciplinarily and conceptually – and the tone inclusively multivocal so as to represent the complex and interwoven ways that ideas about, and culturally constructed practices of, time interrelate with personal sensations and experiences of time.

Through focusing on time and the temporal in performer training, the book offers innovative ways of integrating research into studio practices. Integration, that is, arising from blurring the boundaries between the historic and the contemporary, between collective and individual or professional and amateur practices that are evident synchronously within training. The range of research interests explored includes ideas on age/aging and children in the training context, how training impacts over a lifetime, the duration of training and the impact of training regimes over time, concepts of timing and the 'right' time, how time is viewed from a range of international training perspectives, the intersections of amateur, festival, digital and institutionalized time with training, and taking the long view on collectives, ensembles and fashions in training, their decay or endurance. The contributors embrace a range of primary identifications, from academic writers and theatre historians to professional artists and practitioner-scholars, while 'performer training' is taken as an umbrella term, inclusive of pedagogies designed for actors, physical theatre performers, dancers, and classical and folk singers. The aim has been to include a wide range of perspectives to provide a platform for further interdisciplinary engagement and debate in this rich but under-researched terrain. For this reason, the volume includes full-length chapters, shorter essays and provocations and many illustrations divided into five sections.

The opening section, 'About Time: Narratives of Time,' is concerned with ways in which the temporality of performer training is rendered narratable and how time is narrativized through performer-training practices. Remembering, historicizing, marketing or, even, talking about training, all can establish or challenge potent frameworks around the training experience. Mark Evans seeks to explore how the personal narrative of training evades and disrupts chronological time. His writing reflects on the ways that various time planes and experiences of time can coexist or intersect, rendering the notion of lineage palpable. David Wiles' provocation piece seeks to interrupt accepted timeframes of modern(ist) actor training and draw our attention to longer timescales and to histories of performer training that have been obscured by the drive of 20th-century systematization. Evi Stamatiou's chapter argues for a rethinking of the commodification of time in conservatoire training through the engagement of a feminist chronopolitics. She explores the risks for women in investing time in actor training in relation to their prospects for future employment. Diego Pellecchia and Udaka Tatsushige critically reflect on the training of Noh Theatre performers, who are learning within the context of Japanese traditional practices that are inextricably linked to the notion of time and its passing. The training of Noh performers is divided into phases prescribed by tradition, and can span from early childhood until the student's mid-20s. As one of the great theorists of Noh, Zeami Motokiyo (c. 1363–c. 1443), noted, each age has its 'flower' of performance.

The next section, 'On Time: Temporalizing Time through Technique,' explores how particular techniques and technical challenges offer us insights into the experience of time, and how time and temporality interweave with the development and practice of technique. Darren Tunstall's chapter looks at the notion of good timing and unpicks what lies behind this idea, asking where we get the belief in a sense of timing from and how we might train actors to improve their timing. After considering the historical shifts in definitions of timing, he introduces the psychological concepts which reveal that timing is not merely subjective, but rather has socially shared features and underpinning neurological principles. He places timing as a central feature of social relations and argues the extent to which our sense of time is subject to environmental constraints that allow for a dynamic ecology of timing. Jenny Swingler's provocation takes the Twenty Movements, a central feature of the first year in the Lecoq training, and examines the exercise as an invitation for students to trace the steps of this exercise's past while embodying it in the present. She takes this experience and considers how it can become of use to her journey as a performer. In South Indian contexts, training is a practice in itself; Mark Hamilton's chapter explores his experience of time through his own training in the *adavu* (core drills) of *bharatanatyam* (South Indian classical dance). He argues that in this context, calendrical time is challenged by rhythms and temporal patterns of movement that infuse immediate physical existence with spiritual experiences that extend beyond the present moment such that past, present and future can merge into each other. This creates particular challenges for the trainee performer, that he examines from the perspective of a Western student. The section finishes with a chapter by Gyllian Raby in which she takes the 'wicked problems' and the time pressures involved in devising theatre, and considers the ways in which Anna and Lawrence Halprin's RSVP cycles (Resources, Scores, eValuative analysis/ Valuaction and Performance) enable performers/devisers to sidestep such anxieties. The different temporalities possible within the cycles of the RSVP process can positively affect the experiences of devisers and settle the anxieties typical to the conventional theatre production process.

Section three, 'Over Time: Age, Duration, Longevity,' questions ways in which training endures over time, whether renewed and revalued within each maturing artist performer or through a form of training practice that is sufficiently malleable so as to be able to surf time. In this series of chapters, authors examine training methods that resist apparent limitations determined by age or traditions, to reveal revitalized attitudinal approaches, working methods and skills acquirement that surface only with an open, fluid understanding of longevity and age. For his essay on Carnatic singing and young trainees, Tim Jones interviews Indu, the daughter of his first teacher, K. R. Sivasankara Panikkar, who is also now a teacher. Rather than using age as the sole definitional characteristic of youth, Jones merges the childhood of his teacher, his daughter, her trainees and his own early training experiences in Carnatic music as an adult to talk about the childhood *of* training itself, a childhood renewed across generations. Tiffany Strawson reflects on her own and other women's experience of traditional training for *topeng*, the Balinese Masked-Dance drama. Using the critical lens of 'new interculturalism,' she explores how culturally specific temporalities impact and nuance the experience of performer training in Bali, with specific reference to the aging body within the context of a training system that embraces repetition and endurance. What happens when 'something at the heart' of your practice goes dead? As a mature ballet dancer and choreographer, this question prompted Jennifer Jackson to return to studio practice working with teacher Roger Tully. In this provocation, she considers how ballet teaching based on his concept, that each dancer 'has the ideal body for their own dance,' offers fresh perspectives applicable for mature and younger dancers. For instance, Jackson re-examines ballet principles, such as the use of 'aplomb,' through the analysis of their subtle temporal states. In the final chapter within the segment, Jane Turner and Patrick Campbell focus on the ways in which time shapes and is manifest within the training processes of three artists: Luis Alonso, Carolina Pizarro and Mia Theil Have. All three are exponents of Third Theatre, defined by the authors as a 'multifarious, transnational entity, comprised of groups and solo artists across the world' who typically take training and a laboratory environment as essential to their practice. Through the application of Deleuze's fluid mapping of 'becomings' rather than a more fixed sense of 'being' to the selected artists' practices, they substitute ideas of linear time progression in individual training and lineages with a more active approach. This involves changeability, ruptures and regeneration, all of which offer a better fit for discussing Third Theatre.

The fourth section of the book, 'Out of Time: Beyond Presence and the Present,' tackles the notion of 'the present' as a recurrent and aspirational quality of performer training and examines its unruly multiplicity and possibilities. The opening chapter extends the examination of Third Theatre practices and investigates the training developed by the Bridge of Winds. Over the last 30 years, the company of international artists meets annually for a training residency, its members then continuing the training in their respective countries and with their own companies. What brings these artists back to a training, the core principles of which have remained the same, and how is this long-term present experienced as both continually unfolding and intermittent? In search of an answer, Adriana La Selva draws on Deleuze's theorization of repetition and unpacks its implications for the ethos of the company's work. The chapter by Konstantinos Thomaidis interweaves interviews with voice practitioners, findings in voice science and micro-phenomenological analysis to listen closely to a crucial 'moment' in training: the simultaneous act of voicing and listening to oneself while voicing. Challenging perceived understandings of vocal presence, the chapter rethinks the timespace of voicing as a continuum from idiotopic endochrony to allotopic exochrony and makes a case for the potential of a disruptive voice pedagogy. Laura Vorwerg's essay reframes the interdisciplinary demands placed upon contemporary performers as an issue linked to embodied temporality (the moment at which a trained performer arrives at another discipline) but also to the monetization of production time (time allowed during rehearsals to acquire new skills). Using examples from recent theatre and opera performances, Vorwerg proposes three ways of dealing with the temporal conundrum posed by interdisciplinarity: selective skill development, collaborative disciplinary integration and collaborative skill augmentation. Chan E. Park's essay displaces the present even further through its examination of *pansori*, a Korean sung narrative tradition. Since its designation as intangible cultural heritage, *pansori* performance has become a 'time capsule': the form, vocal style and repertoire of the genre were crystallized in the 19th century before its decline in popularity in the first half of the 20th century, but singers are now called to engage contemporary and transnational audiences. Which training techniques are, then, essential to the contemporary performer of *pansori*?

In the final section, 'From Time to Times: Expansive Temporalities,' the volume steps out beyond the more traditional places of training to open up the issue of time in relation to contested training practices that take place online (Massive Open Online Courses, MOOCs, for instance), in festival spaces, while socializing and in folk or amateur practices. Jonathan Pitches opens his chapter by noting the degree to which performer training continues to extend its online presence and, while this can be seen as a potential challenge to studio transmission, he assesses the potential advantages it can offer through 'its mix of synchronous and asynchronous modes of learning.' Pitches takes his experiences of running MOOCs with their paradoxical relationship to both 'eventness' and existence in perpetuity, as the springboard for an examination of the ways that 'time is uniquely organized in digital performer training.' From a very different perspective, Kate Craddock also appreciates the significance of online interaction and networking, in her case, as a means of nurturing festival participants' experience beyond the event. Founder and Festival Director of GIFT (Gateshead International Festival of Theatre) in North East England, Craddock investigates the impact of festival 'time out of time.' The magnified temporal experiences of festival time can, she argues, disorientate participants to a degree that positively supports opening up to interaction across national, age, experience and disciplinary boundaries. The corollary of this, she suggests, is further potential for training found both in the festival workshop/performance times and in their interstices. Eugénie Pastor, a founder member of the theatre company Little Bulb, offers a provocation that uncovers an unusual training terrain. Developed to suit the idiosyncratic style of Little Bulb's devised performances, Pastor asserts that neither she nor the other seven members of the company, are formally trained. They learned 'their craft through spending a lot of time doing it.' In this instance, therefore, training time leeches into all-time, just as the group's professional working lives interweave with their social friendships. She describes this 'collective intimacy' as the instigator of artistic training with concomitant impact on their experience of time and performance-making. The final chapter in the section, by Libby Worth, contains resonances with all three that precede it as Worth considers the nature of dance training in folk and traditional dance forms. Using case-study examples of clog and rapper sword dancing practices happening in London, she examines how historic choreographies, dance materials (clogs and rapper swords) and narratives drawn from an industrial heritage remain both present and altered in contemporary dance practice. Observation of the all-female dance side (group), the Tower Ravens Rapper, uncovers the ways in which dancers are able to negotiate the extensive dance traditions with their current interests and concerns through virtuosic technique acquired in leisure time.

Collectively, the contributions to the volume ask questions such as:

- Do training regimes have their own lifespan? What might newness, maturity and decrepitude mean for a training regime? How might we usefully compare old and new training regimes?
- How does training work its effects on the body over time? How important is time in the changes that training initiates? How important is time for the training process and how much time do we need to train?
- Timing in performance can be determined: counts, music, breath rhythms or open improvisational response. How are these different approaches accounted for within training? What does 'good timing' mean and can it be taught?
- How training relates to age, how training itself ages and how time relates to notions of maturity, experience, decay, decline, birth and death within the context of training, its practices and its histories? How is training renewed, recycled or revisited? Does training itself have an age?
- What is the duration of training, the experience of time during training and the timing of training activity? At what age might training begin or end? How might training be differently inflected for older or younger trainees? Can and indeed should children be trained for performance? At what age might training stop? How might training change throughout the lifespan of a performer? How do training collectives, ensembles and institutions experience and negotiate change, aging or renewal?
- Do the changes of the body and voice over time offer challenges and opportunities for the trainee and the trainer? How do the temporalities of imagination, memory, cognition, sensuality and perception correlate with physio-vocal temporalities?
- How important is the rhythm of training? What can best be learnt slowly and what can best be learnt at speed? When and why is training experienced as an intensity of time, and when as a loosening of time? In an age where time = money and in which time is increasingly foreshortened, what might be the value of taking one's time, and is such a process a luxury or a necessity? Can we speed up training? What forms of resistance to preconceived understandings of time, speed and velocity can training propose?

The trajectory proposed by the structure of the book, while not exhaustive or conclusive, is indicative of our intention to move past a single or unified approach to the temporality of training. As the following chapters attest, personal memories from one's time in training evoke new histories of training. These, in turn, frame the way trainees narrate their own history to themselves, and these narratives are not only chronological accounts but also a means to place value upon one's life-story. Techniques and practices temporalize time, rendering it into felt experiences of rhythm, tempo, repetition and timing, while the longevity of some practices witnesses the duration, aging and renewal of training itself. The present of training may integrate its phenomenal pasts and futures beyond linear causality or include returns to the precise moment of an exercise after year-long intervals. Shifting and emergent contexts of training – digital and amateur, among others – may expand the temporality of training beyond synchronous co-presence in the studio or divisions between professional and nonprofessional timeframes. In conjoining time and training in multiple and unexpected ways, the expansive temporalities of training discussed across the book position peda-gogy as agential in the sociocultural temporalization of the performer, and time in training as an issue compellingly urgent and elusively unresolved.

In this light, we wish to conclude this Introduction and open *Time and Per-former Training* with a final set of questions directly addressed to our readers:

- How do you experience time and temporality in your training?
- How do the various practices and cross-disciplinary discussions of time in the following chapters connect with your training needs and experiences?
- In what ways can you use the above list of questions as additional provoca-tions that you may wish to take up within your own training practice, as either student or teacher?
- In other words, how can the temporality of reading a book about training be rethought as *training time*?

Notes

1 Phelan, in her latest work, also proposed a more multifaceted nexus of temporal connec-tions between performance, documentation and history (2010, 2014). More recently, Laura Cull's writing has continued and extended the critical interrogation of presence at the junctures of performance and philosophy. Her work on Deleuze, in particular, has advocated that performance can not only represent time differently' or make audiences conscious 'of the idea that life operates at multiple speeds' but, more importantly, allow 'the multiplicity of duration to be something *lived*, rather than merely contemplated or reflected on from a safe distance' (Cull 2012: 179; original emphasis).
2 And the list can now include Wickstrom's just-published *Fiery Temporalities* (2018).
3 For a useful cross-disciplinary summation of trends within the temporal turn, see Hassan (2010). The first chapter in Christine Ross's monograph maps the cross-fertilization of time studies, the temporal turn and research in the Humanities, Arts and Social Sciences (2012: 18–52).
4 The debate is heavily inflected by Kant's unresolved presentation of time as both internal sense and external/*a priori*/formal condition as well as the Bergsonian differ-entiation between clock time as abstraction and lived time as real duration. Excel-lent synopses of, and interventions in, relevant debates can be found in Ross (2012: 18–52), Jakovljevic (2014) and Grant et al. (2015: 3–11). Such distinction between time and temporality implicitly underpins the discussion of 'objective, external time' and 'subjective, internal time' by Pavis (2003: 155–59).

References

Auslander, P. (2008) *Liveness: Performance in a Mediatized Culture*, New York: Routledge.
Carlson, M. (2001) *The Haunted Stage: The Theatre as Memory Machine*, Ann Arbor: Uni-versity of Michigan Press.

Cull, L. (2009) *Differential Presence: Deleuze and Performance*, Ph.D. thesis, Exeter, Devon: University of Exeter.

———— (2012) *Theatres of Immanence: Deleuze and the Ethics of Performance*, Basingstoke: Palgrave Macmillan.

Ellis, S.T. (2013) *Doing the Time Warp: Queer Temporalities and Musical Theater*, Ph.D. thesis, Los Angeles, CA: UCLA.

Evans, M. (2009) *Movement Training for the Modern Actor*, New York and Oxon: Routledge.

Grant, S., McNeilly, N. and Veerapen, M. (eds) (2015) *Performance and Temporalisation: Time Happens*, Basingstoke: Palgrave.

Hassan, R. (2010) 'Globalization and the "temporal turn": recent trends and issues in time studies,' *The Korean Journal of Policy Studies*, 25(2): 83–102.

Jakovljevic, B. (2014) 'Editorial: now then – performance and temporality: not once, not twice…,' *Performance Research*, 20(5): 1–8.

Jakovljevic, B. and Mantoan, L. (eds) (2014) *On Time: Special Issue of Performance Research*, 19(3).

Kartsaki, E. and Schmidt, T. (eds) (2015) *On Repetition: Special Issue of Performance Research*, 20(5).

Kelly, D. (2015) *Time in Early Modern English Theatre and Culture*, Ph.D. thesis, Belfast: Queen's University Belfast.

Lehmann, H.-T. (2006) *Postdramatic Theatre*, New York and Oxon: Routledge.

Limon, J. (2010) *The Chemistry of Theatre: Performativity of Time*, Basingstoke: Palgrave.

————. (2014) 'Time in theatre,' in Reynolds, B. (ed.) *Performance Studies: Key Words, Concepts and Theories*, Basingstoke: Palgrave Macmillan, 215–26.

Manninen, S.L.A. (2014) *Duration Materialised: Investigating Contemporary Performance as a Temporal Medium*, Ph.D. thesis, London: Queen Mary.

Pavis, P. (2003) *Analyzing Performance: Theater, Dance, and Film*, transl. D. Williams, Ann Arbor: University of Michigan Press.

Phelan, P. (1993) *Unmarked: The Politics of Performance*, New York: Routledge.

————. (2010) 'Haunted stages: performance and the photographic effect,' in Blessing, J. (ed.) *Haunted: Contemporary Photography/Video/Performance*, New York: Guggenheim Museum, 50–87.

————. (2014) 'On the difference between time and history,' *Performance Research*, 19(3): 114–19.

Rabey, D.I. (2016) *Theatre, Time and Temporality: Melting Clocks and Snapped Elastics*, Chicago, IL: University of Chicago Press.

Ross, C. (2012) *The Past Is the Present; It's the Future too: The Temporal Turn in Contemporary Art*, London and New York: Continuum.

Scheer, E. (ed.) (2012) *On Duration: Special Issue of Performance Research*, 17(5).

Schneider, R. (2011) *Performing Remains: Art and War in Times of Theatrical Reenactment*, New York: Routledge.

————. (2014) *Theatre & History*, Basingstoke: Palgrave Macmillan.

Senior, A. and The Institute for the Art and Practice of Dissent at Home. (eds) (2018) *On Children: Special Issue of Performance Research*, 23(1).

Taylor, D. (2003) *The Archive and the Repertoire: Performing Cultural Memory in the Americas*, Durham: Duke UP.

Wagner, M. (2012) *Shakespeare, Theatre and Time*, New York: Routledge.

Wakefield, N. (2016) *Performing Temporalities: A Practice-based Pursuit of Time-specificity Drawing on the Philosophy of Henri Bergson and the Performances of Tehching Hsieh, Every House Has a Door, Janez Janša, Janez Janša and Janez Janša*, Ph.D. thesis, London: RHUL.

Wickstrom, M. (2016) 'Thinking about temporality and theatre,' *The Journal of American Drama and Theatre*, 28(1), http://jadtjournal.org/2016/03/23/thinking-about-temporality-and-theatre/.

———. (2018) *Fiery Temporalities in Theatre and Performance*, London: Bloomsbury.

Wiles, D. (2014) *Theatre & Time*, Basingstoke: Palgrave Macmillan.

Zarrilli, P. (1990) 'What does it mean to "become the character": power, presence, and transcendence in Asian in-body disciplines of practice,' in Schechner, R. and Appel, W. (eds) *By Means of Performance: Interculutral Studies of Theatre and Ritual*, Cambridge: Cambridge University Press, 131–48.

SECTION II
About time
Narratives of time

3

LECOQ

Training, time and temporality

Mark Evans

20 December 2017 (Coventry)

It will be five or ten years before you understand the training you will begin today.

(Evans, notes from Jacques Lecoq's address to new students,
11 October 1982)

Thirty-three years on.

I have met with so many fellow ex-students. Our conversations, memories and reflections continue to tumble through my embodied consciousness, creating a web of images, impressions, actions and movements – all linked through time and all changing through time. The School, one place and one time, but linking so many other places and moments, has built for me an embodied sense of the rhythms of theatre, time, training, making, thinking and writing.

All training starts and ends at some point in time, and all training lasts for a certain period of time – however brief or long, however fragmented or flexible. Theatre training also divides time: into before, during and after; into different classes or sessions; and into choices taken or not taken. Training additionally works to enable the theatrically effective use of time – for the performer and for the audience – through selection, refinement and manipulation. Like time, training is demarcated by critical moments of change and transformation. Like time, it also deals in repetition and the rhythmic dynamics of repetition. My training is a personal experience of a shared phenomenon, similar to my experiences of time.

Training sets forward the bringing forth of what was immanent in the student-performer. Merleau-Ponty writes, 'A past and a future spring forth when I reach out towards them' (2000: 421) – much theatre training encourages the students to bring forward to consciousness the experience of their pasts, and to project themselves forward towards the person and performer that they seek to be, framed within a particular period of time, a particular historical context and its cultural needs. Training regimes therefore are deeply involved in the making of important cultural decisions – whether to develop the student's ability to reach forward through time towards the performer that they might become, or to develop a student who accepts the impact of a training regime at a certain point in time on their embodied selves, as part of their professionalization.

I reach back…

11 October 1982 (École Jacques Lecoq, Paris)

> École Jacques Lecoq, 9.00am. I'm up early because I don't know how long it'll take. When I arrive – chaos! People still registering and paying.
>
> Then after waiting together for maybe ¾ hour Lecoq comes to tell us about the course. […] Everyone seems a little uncertain, but happy to be here.
>
> It is a 'journey,' he says, 'work we undertake together…' What am I trying to find – is it to learn about theatre or about myself, I wonder which I will learn more about.

(Evans 1983)

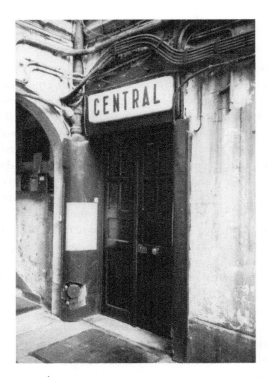

FIGURE 3.1 Le Central, École Jacques Lecoq, 1982. Photo: Mark Evans.

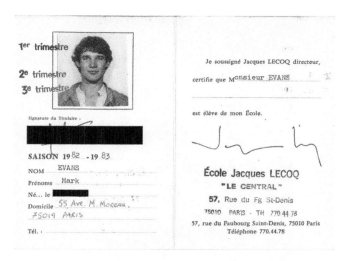

FIGURE 3.2 *Carte étudiant*, 1982–1983.

Time at the Lecoq School is a form of distance travelled, a series of changes and transformations, meetings and departures (Figure 3.1 and 3.2). As students, we are all starting from the moment before the training begins, coming together unaware of the experiences yet to come and only half aware of the experiences that have shaped us and brought us to this place and this time. For one year or two, we are together as a class, and then we become former students and begin from then onwards to measure our time apart and our time away from the School.

At the end of our time as students, we will leave – to make work, to make sense of the training in the context outside the School, to continue the process of making sense of ourselves.

16 July 2015 (École internationale de théâtre Jacques Lecoq, Paris)

11.00 am. I am returning to the School a little over 15 years after Jacques Lecoq's death and 32 years after I finished as a student Figure 3.3. I am meeting with two of his children, his daughter Pascale and his son Richard. I walk past the photos of past students in the hallway – people I remember from my own year, their young faces smiling out at me. The many faces of students from subsequent years, a reminder of the time that has passed, each set of photos marking out another year.

> People who know me and whom I have not seen for a long time often ask: 'So what do you do now?' I reply, 'The school!' I see disappointment in the eyes of my interrogators and a lack of enthusiasm when confronted by my reply. 'You still teach?' 'Yes, every day, as long as there are still students'.
>
> *(Lecoq 1996 [2016]: 273, author's translation)*

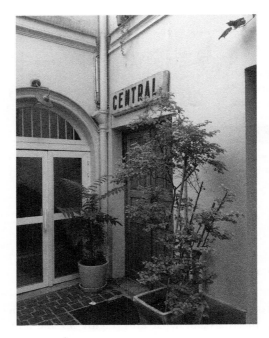

FIGURE 3.3 Le Central, L'École Internationale de Théâtre Jacques Lecoq, 2015. Photo: Mark Evans.

Pascale describes how her mother, Fay, wanted to upgrade the *grande salle* after Jacques' death. Pascale prefers it renovated, but visibly the same; the history still living in the fabric of the room. It is still very much as I remember it – I can feel my body wanting to move through the *grande salle* again, sensing its generous length, breadth and height. When I visit the School, it is always fascinating to catch glimpses of students working on familiar exercises. There is no sense of anything fixed in time, instead a patient process of evolution and change that is a response to each new set of students. As I watch, I am aware of the experience of time flowing around me, and the exercises that we have shared act as the river banks that shape that flow.

The training process in the first year does not feel like a process of embellishment, of the student acquiring a set of predefined skills. Instead the training requires the student to recognize and then to attempt to let go of what they already know. The exercises and the structure of the training are deceptively simple. This simplicity enables each part of the training to be remade at an individual level by each student and to be revisited in various ways at various stages. In this sense, the training can remain virtually unchanged and yet still be remade by the students each year.

The training both matures and endures – simple but powerful points of reference that students and graduates come back to again and again in their work.

When former students gather and wherever they gather, it seems to be common that at some point they return to their experience of some of these exercises that they share across the years. Despite the students' individual experience, the exercises seem to function very effectively as shared reference points through time.

18 October 1982 (École Jacques Lecoq, Paris)

I am 24. The School requires students to have previous experience – but although experience is required, it feels like it is also a liability, something that can hold you back, trip you over. Resilience is important, a certain determination and commitment to see things through and to survive the knocks, and the playfulness to keep the training in perspective. The inescapable hurdle in the first term is to make the 'cut' before Christmas, when around a quarter of the students learn that they will not be coming back next term. The possibility of failure makes time feel precious. Time, age and experience writ too heavily on the body make the experience of the School harder and potentially more fragile. There is an urgency to achieve, succeed, make progress and to survive – this keeps students in the moment of their training and pushes them forward into new experiences that they do not yet know how to conceptualize.

14 July 1983 (London)

I am back in the UK, looking for work. I audition; directors look puzzled as I explain how we explored 'fire' as an element. I realize that this training, my trained body and what it can now do, is ahead of its time. I realize that despite the roots that it has connecting with the work of Jacques Copeau[1] in the 1920s, it is a training more innovative and more profoundly contemporary than most conventional actor-training regimes in the 1980s, fulfilling Jacques' aim that the school should 'produce a young theatre of new work' so that 'each student will go on to make his (*sic*) own journey using the foundations we provide' (Lecoq 2002: 16).

As I start my own journey as a teacher, later in the 1980s, I move from using my knowledge towards understanding my knowledge. This trajectory takes me from my experience of making work in the present back to the past of my training in Paris and then forward to the future of the students I teach. I also realize how it is that the teacher stands still while the students move on, and how the teacher gets older while the students stay young.

22 January 1999 (Coventry)

I read in *The Guardian* newspaper that Lecoq has died. The memories flood back. Now I am in a different time – a time after Jacques Lecoq. After Lecoq. I consider what that means – something different for me than for those who have studied at the School after 1999? The early 1980s was a time in my life that was and will always be inhabited by Jacques Lecoq and by the teachers and students at the School at that time. The School that continues now without Jacques passes on the experience of his presence without the presence itself – and it successfully continues to function in this way. It succeeds by building on Jacques' own awareness of the need both to evolve in response to the changing times and also repeatedly to present the student with fixed challenges that the students know have been repeated by many cohorts of students over many years.

> I always thought that the students didn't need teachers in order to be of their time and that we, the teachers, needed rather to provide the permanent reference points.
>
> *(Lecoq 1996 [2016]: 273, author's translation)*

15 July 2015 (Paris)

Evening. It's very hot tonight. The tenth *arrondissement* is alive with families squabbling and Arab, Asian and North African men talking on the streets. The *quartier* around the School, always a busy working area of the city, has now become a chic evening destination! Soaking in the dynamics of the *quartier*, I remember that the *auto-cours* process, in which students devise their own responses to themes set by the tutors, is one of the elements that allow the outside in and link the course to its specific time and place and in subtle ways to its historical context, bringing the changes of the times into the classroom. At the end of the first year, this process is most completely embodied in the extended task given to the students, *les enquêtes*,[2] in which students are tasked to research a milieu and then to create a performance that encapsulates the qualities of that milieu for a public audience. Through this process, as the city changes the School changes with it.

November 1982 (École Jacques Lecoq, Paris)

In the changing rooms and in the local bar (*Chez Jeanette*), we share stories we have heard of past students, and of changes to the course – the start of the *auto-cours*, the improvisation theme of the journey across the city becoming an *auto-cours*, the arrival of the clown as a dramatic territory in the second year. We become aware of how Lecoq is responding to us and to what we offer him, of how our changing interests and abilities over time are the lifeblood of the School.

Later, I stand in the corridor between the *salle verte* and the student changing rooms while a fellow student uses my camera to take my photograph (Figure 3.4).

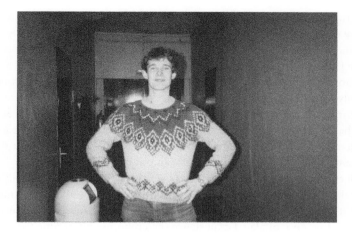

FIGURE 3.4   Mark Evans, corridor of École Jacques Lecoq, 1982.

16 July 2015 (École internationale de théâtre Jacques Lecoq, Paris)

I stand in the same corridor thirty-three years later, while Richard Lecoq, Jacques and Fay's son, takes my photograph. I know that my body has changed but it still remembers so much. Years of observing bodies in movement, of moving, and of training my own body and those of others – my body remembers what is the same, but it also remembers the differences. Exercises repeated over and over, and across decades. Lecoq used to say to us, 'Move while your knees still let you!' Then I laughed, now I smile (Figure 3.5).

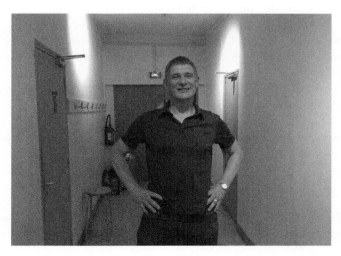

FIGURE 3.5   Mark Evans, corridor of École Jacques Lecoq, 2015.

The immediate effects of the training on my younger body were to enlarge my sense of space – '*jouer plus grand*.' I had always been nimble, but the training helped me to become more precise, more confident and also to find playfulness in what I did and to value its qualities. I struggled with handstands and some of the more advanced acrobatics. I sustained a muscular injury, which curtailed my involvement in some of the classes for a few weeks – I learned to watch and observe instead. Living in Paris on little money and using my body every day meant that I lost weight and gained muscle tone. I noted with some pleasure that these changes in my body matched equally in my increased ability to observe movement and in my general confidence in physical improvisation.

I reflect on the effects of the training over time; the deposits that the training has laid down. How it endures over time in my body – how quickly and easily I can call it back. Yet the changes in my body mean that my energy has changed along with my sense of play. I experience the embodiment of time through these changes.

Now I am also an academic, I write about and research the work of Lecoq and also the work of one of his pedagogic predecessors, Jacques Copeau. I am aware that what has become embodied in me also has a history of its own. The systematically trained body as a phenomenon and as a process is also ageing – it is no longer the fresh innovation that it was in the early part of the 20th century, and yet every new student discovers this training all afresh despite the School's celebration of its sixtieth birthday, all the publications that capture and reflect on Lecoq's pedagogy and the availability of information about Lecoq on the internet.

Weds 8 June 1983 (École Jacques Lecoq, Paris)

Final feedback from the tutors before I leave:

> 'Didn't play enough. Doubt myself too often. Lots of talent. First term good (others not so good). Work with words, in a troupe. Many things expected.'
> 'Good sense of timing in the theatre – able to taste a moment well. Good with words. Some very good things – real surprises.'
> 'Good and stable – need to work on moving weight. Very good "20 movements." Capable of much more than I think I am. Impose myself more in the space.'

16 July 2015 (Coventry)

I could feel my body changing during the training – an increased mastery of movement, greater confidence in acrobatics, a heightened awareness of where I am in space and the dynamics of my movement. This is a set of changes enabled by the work with the neutral mask – exercises that many students have performed before and after me, and yet the results of which are now distinctively my own.

Now, at a greater distance from the training I feel a different mastery – one of custom and habit, of familiarity, understanding and ingrained practice. Well beyond the need to remember the exercises, I have become more alert to their resonances, significances and reverberations. Lecoq writes about his hope that the training will allow students 'to be consummate livers of life' (2002: 16). The implication, which I feel now to be true, is that the training becomes part of the way in which life is lived – you grow from the neutral mask being something that is worn during training towards the neutral mask being a deep and profound part of how you understand the world in which you live.

October 1982 – July 2015 (Paris and London)

28 October 1982 – *La Chambre d'Enfance* (The Childhood Room) – rediscover a room that you knew as a child. Find the right moment to move through time and return/revisit the experience of childhood. Not exactly the re-enactment of a precise memory or moment in time, but an improvised performance of the experience of time – what is the quality of that moment when you become the child again. The exercise can be easily misunderstood as psychological – it is not; it is deeply physical.

10 July 2015 – I am talking with Ayse Tashkiran, a former Lecoq student and now a tutor at Royal Central School of Speech and Drama. She recalls that for her, animal work was about being right in the present tense, very different from the more epic timescale of the neutral mask.

3 November 1982 – *Le Village* (The Village) – our *auto-cours* theme, twenty-four hours in the life of a village condensed into fifteen minutes, the whole class working together. Which moments pass quickly and which pass slowly – creating theatrical time, encapsulating time?

10 July 2015 – Ayse remembers the experience of acrobatics, caught in timeless moments of holding a handstand, throwing herself through a backflip. Timing and timelessness. We talk about how the neutral mask creates time for you, opens up time and timing as something physical, something understood through the body. The fundamental journey, an exercise through several environments undertaken in the neutral mask, also takes place over time, from dawn to dusk.

12 November 1982 – *The Fundamental Journey: From the Forest to the Mountain.* Lecoq says, 'Take time. Impose your creation on the time, the silence, by your immobility. Learn to feel what the audience feels as the right time – the collective feel' (Evans 1983).

Weds 1 June 1983 (École Jacques Lecoq, Paris)

Gestures, actions and movements all have a beginning, middle and end. Some also repeat. I think about the twenty movements. Actions such as the discus throw – a complete action launching intention into the future – and the *grande godille* – endlessly sculling through the water, beginning and ending in continuous

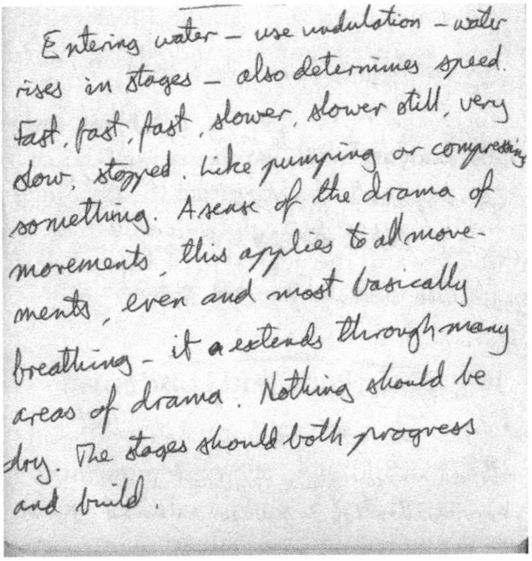
Entering water – use undulation – water
rises in stages – also determines speed.
Fast, fast, fast, slower, slower still, very
slow, stopped. Like pumping or compressing
something. A sense of the drama of
movements, this applies to all movements, even and most basically
breathing – it a extends through many
areas of drama. Nothing should be
dry. The stages should both progress
and build.

FIGURE 3.6 Extract from Evans (1983).

repetition. Each movement teaching the dynamics of time and space and opening up my body to the rhythms of movement (Figure 3.6).

18 June 2011 (Clore Learning Centre (RSC), Stratford-upon-Avon)

RSC fiftieth Birthday events – I deliver a workshop on the chorus work of Michel Saint-Denis[3]. Referencing Lecoq's work on chorus, I ask a group of acting students to try and balance the stage like a plateau. The actor Clifford Rose, one of the original 1962 RSC ensemble members, recalls Saint-Denis using the same exercise. Suddenly the history of the exercise and its roots through the work of Copeau, Suzanne Bing,[4] Saint-Denis, Jean Dasté[5] and Lecoq become real and tangible. History is present in the room, through movement. I experience the physical way in which training exercises are adapted over time, passing down through different sets of hands.

What does the age of an exercise mean? Training is a pragmatic process and exercises only have currency in so far as they are useful in the now – teachers typically defer the history till after the experience is over. In so far as we do experience the history of exercises, I puzzle as to how this can function not as a hindrance but as something that might enrich the students' learning. It is important to realize that exercises have been made and do have various cultural histories embedded in and circulating around them. Acknowledging this fact also enables the student to understand how they might begin to make their own pedagogy. This was a process that Lecoq himself undertook during the time he worked in Italy. He studied the traditions and techniques of commedia dell'arte, before developing his own approach to improvised masked performance that made sense for his own students and the context of his time. This was a process he then replicated for classical tragedy, melodrama, clowning, *bouffons* and *pantomime blanche*. Whilst Lecoq never belittled the deeper history of the exercises he taught, he realized that some students found it difficult, even without the history being explicitly raised, to move beyond feelings of reverence for some of the forms. For some graduates, this reverence will even transfer to the exercises devised by Lecoq himself – work with the neutral mask, for instance, might be taught with a reverence (rather than respect) that Lecoq would surely have found inimical to his pedagogic aims.

May 1982 (Berkhamsted)

The Lecoq School brochure arrives from Paris.
'The school is intended for persons of a certain maturity who have finished their studies' (École Jacques Lecoq, information sheet, 1982).
When is the right time to go? What is 'a certain maturity'? Have I finished my studies?
I realize that I will only know by going. The right time is now.

3 January 1983 (École Jacques Lecoq, Paris)

'Three people up, have to improvise colours as given by Lecoq. How long do colours 'last'. Red – quick, dense. Blue – long. Green – difficult' (Evans 1983).

Rhythm and timing seem to be integral to all of the training in the first year at the School. There are a number of questions that I keep coming back to:

When is an exercise over?
When has it begun?
When is the right time for an action, gesture, entrance?
How long should a scene last?
What are the differences between time for the group and time for the individual?
When is training over?

10 July 2015 (London)

Ayse and I remember how Lecoq would stop an exercise or an *auto-cours* if the rhythm, energy or breath had already faded away or missed its moment. Sometimes an improvisation was finished before it had started – 'c'est déjà finis.' Sometimes students finished too early, just as the work was starting to develop. Sometimes they went on too long. Even a gesture – the lifting of an arm – has its own timing and dynamics, and its own beginning, middle and end. The training seeks to extend this subtle and detailed understanding into the making of theatre, and even the living of life.

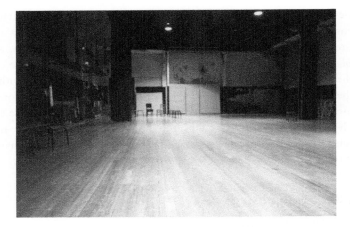

FIGURE 3.7 La Grande Salle, École Jacques Lecoq, 1982. Photo: Mark Evans.

11 October 1982 (École Jacques Lecoq, Paris)

The first *auto-cours* theme – a place and an event. What counts as an event? When is a moment significant and why? What happens in a space that makes an event have meaning? How do we create that moment, not as an individual or a number of individuals, but as a group? What brings a group together in a moment of time to create an event? What is immanent within the space we work in, within when we are working and within who we are singly and together? What happens when the event is finished? (Figure 3.7).

11 August 2015 (Coventry)

I understand now that moving and stopping – balance and imbalance – create both space *and* time.

Lecoq frequently referred to fixed points. The points around which movement happened and which in effect, defined the movement as movement. I realize that fixed points can also be moments in time – points around which events circulate and take their meaning.

The different 'styles' of theatre that are explored in the second year of the School are of course not historically fixed reference points, they are not used as historically defined periods of practice, but as 'dramatic territories'.

11 October 1982 (École Jacques Lecoq, Paris)

The day starts at 2.00 pm for our group. We have one hour of either *préparation corporelle*, movement analysis or acrobatics. Then one and a half hours of improvisation class, followed by one and half hours of *auto-cours* time. Every Wednesday classes stop for the sharing of the *auto-cours* presentations. This cycle of activity

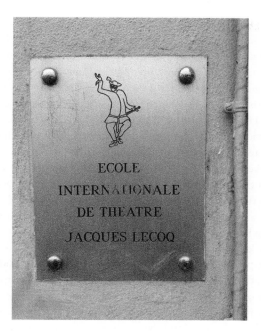

FIGURE 3.8 École internationale de théâtre Jacques Lecoq, 57, rue du faubourg
St. Denis, Paris 75010, 16 July 2015. Photo: Mark Evans.

becomes familiar and shapes the patterns of our studies – warm-up, prepare the
body, develop technique, create and share. There is both linearity – a sense of
time rolling through a programme of learning – and circularity – patterns and
themes recurring, repeating and transforming.

We are all aware of the formal moments of decision – the end of the first
term (a third of the students rejected), the end of the first year (a third of the
students pass to the second year). Coming and going becomes part of the deeper
rhythms of the School. First years watch the rhythms of the second year from a
distance – their projects and final *commandes* – pondering over their own futures.
Occasionally, the pedagogic year students, or the newer teachers, share anecdotes
with us – bits of School history, their own thoughts and experiences. Increasingly
we are aware of our journey into a community connected over not just years, but
decades. We also have our own moments of decision – whether to jump forward
and volunteer for an improvisation, who else to work with on the *auto-cours*, and
how to interpret the challenges set by Lecoq in the *auto-cours*, *les enquêtes* and *les
commandes*[6] (Figure 3.8).

8 September 2015 (Coventry)

With age comes the realization that in performance-making, my training is no
longer something that I consciously refer to, it just is – it is present in what I do

and how I do it. It is present in my body and I am present in it. However, when I teach, this relationship flips – the effort of the training is visible in the bodies of my students and my own training comes back into my consciousness and into my body as I watch, observe, comment on and engage with the work of the students. My own training no longer just is, it is becoming. The School is a journey through which I realize that I have developed an understanding of myself as an artist and as a performer. Time has continued to deepen the training; the training endures in my body providing me with numerous reminders that I catch myself gathering during my own teaching. Time moves in me. Time moves me. Time moves.

Because of, even as a result of, his death, Lecoq has become a different kind of fixed point than the kind of which he so often spoke in his classes. The training remains as a fulcrum point in time, not a fixed moment but a kind of obstacle or set of challenges around or through which the student has to pass and in doing so discover their own creativity. The teaching remains more or less continuous and consistent, many key exercises have remained essentially the same over several decades. Change happens when the time is ready – the teachers consider such moments carefully, alert to the need to respond to the evolution of the course, and also to recognize the value of the training as a consistent point of reference. The School does not get involved in each student's past or your future – it provides them with the understanding, the techniques and the knowledge for them to do that themselves.

The School/training exists for me as a complex set of embodied memories, events, learning journeys, transitions, leavings and returnings, revisitings and re/memberings (then, re-assembling my sense of my own body; now, putting together the pieces of the past). Writing this chapter has taken me through the traces and echoes of particular moments in time – buildings/rooms, notes, books, photographs (my own as well as those of friends and colleagues and of the School itself), and DVDs.

I look back – seeking to understand what my time during and after Lecoq has given me. It is not the memories and the objects that seem to matter. I realize how much of my training and my experiences time has utterly bound together within me, within the other students that I talk to and across all of us and our experiences. The sharing comes to be so much more important across time than the individual experience.

8 June 1983 and 16 November 2016 (Paris and Coventry)

'Bien. C'est finis.'

Acknowledgements

My thanks to fellow ex-Lecoq School students for the conversations that have stimulated and informed this chapter – in particular, Ayse Tashkiran, Caroline Von Stumm and Malcolm Tulip, for exchanging thoughts, generating ideas and reminding me that memories are better shared.

Notes

1 Jacques Copeau (1879–1949) was a leading figure in the development of French Theatre between the two world wars. A director, actor, playwright and pedagogue, he campaigned passionately for a theatre that was uncluttered and physically expressive. He and his assistant Suzanne Bing are widely credited as the founder figures of modern physical theatre practice (see Evans 2006).
2 *Les enquêtes* are the group tasks set at the end of the first year. Groups identify a milieu that they wish to explore and create a theatrical response to in a first-year performance evening.
3 Michel Saint-Denis was Copeau's nephew and assistant. He founded La Compagnie des Quinze in 1929, and later established significant drama training institutions in the UK, the USA and France. He was one of the initial triumvirate set up to run the Royal Shakespeare Company at its inauguration.
4 Suzanne Bing (1885–1967) was a close associate of Jacques Copeau and collaborated with him as an actress and a teacher. Her work with the School attached to Copeau's Théâtre du Vieux-Colombier provided the foundations for the later development of modern mime (see Evans 2006).
5 Jean Dasté (1904–1994) was a pupil of Jacques Copeau and a core member of the young troupe that Copeau established in Burgundy in 1924, Les Copiaus. He went on to establish his own company after the Second World War, to which, in 1948, he recruited the young Jacques Lecoq as an actor and movement director.
6 *Les commandes* is the name given to the final assignment for the second year students. Each student is given a word or phrase which they can interpret how they wish in the creation of a personal response that will mark their departure from the School.

References

Evans, M. (1983) Private Journal of Studies at Lecoq School, Paris (1982–1983), unpublished.
————. (2006) *Jacques Copeau*, London and New York: Routledge.
Lecoq, J. (1996) *Lettre aux mes élèves*, available in Lecoq, P. (2016) *Jacques Lecoq: un point fixe en mouvement*, Paris: Actes Sud, 272–76.
————. (2002) *The Moving Body: Teaching Creative Theatre*, trans. D. Bradby, London: Bloomsbury.
Merleau-Ponty, M. (2000) *Phenomenology of Perception*, trans. C. Smith, London and New York: Routledge.

4

PREMODERN TRAINING

A provocation

David Wiles

Theatre training did not begin with Stanislavski, though the assumption has become convenient and comfortable because so many people share it. In this brief 'provocation' I shall challenge a continuing modernist obsession with the new, and ask what happened to the classical system of actor training? Why do we still perform the texts of Sophocles, but ignore the wisdom of the past when it comes to acting? Painters and musicians take the premodern world more seriously. Joseph Roach's (1985) *The Player's Passion* is one of the very few serious attempts, at least in English language scholarship, to tackle the history of acting as distinct from the history of actors, but that now influential book hooks the art of acting to the advance of science, allowing us to infer that the theatrical past is of no more practical use today than 18th-century science. So in the first instance, I want to challenge the view of Time's Arrow enshrined in the ideology of progress. Now that the Stanislavski 'system' has had its day, because of commercial pressures on actors to be multiskilled, because in a mediatized age, live theatre needs to redefine itself, and for more complex reasons to do with how we understand ourselves as human beings, it is time to recognize that before Stanislavski, there flourished another great system of acting in Western culture, synthesized by the Roman orator Quintilian (2001) in the 2nd century CE, and repeatedly reworked between the 16th and 19th centuries. Modernism, with its insistence on the new, entailed a significant loss of cultural memory, and I want to suggest that it is time to recall that older system of acting.

The classical system of acting was tied to the art of 'rhetoric,' that is, persuasive public speech, working on the emotions of an audience. And today, speech has effectively been erased from current discourses about actor training, while talk is all of the body, with some acknowledgement of voice. Speech, I want to insist, is also of the body, and connected through processes of evolution to physical gesture. The Romans understood that. By downgrading speech, and allowing it to be confused with the written word, theatre scholars seem to me to negate the principle of psychophysical connectedness that is invoked with such reverence within the discipline. The retreat from speech reflects a loss of faith in public speech within modern democracy. It relates to the great schism mapped out in the Enlightenment between on the one hand emotion, the body and the sphere of the feminine, and on the other hand reason, language and the sphere of the masculine. This schism left no ground where language and the body could meet.

I am currently composing this text on my laptop, for the benefit of unknown readers who will scan these words on a page, or more likely a screen, at some time and place unknown to me. As I sit crouched over my keyboard, I try to re-cover the physical impulse that, nearly two years ago, culminated in ten minutes of energized and gestural speech, as I sought with an appropriate blend of reason and passion to persuade a small group of TaPRA[1] participants of what they must have considered an at best mischievous proposition. My essential idea was bound up with my communicative act. I was able to wave in front of Mark Evans and other participants, a copy of Evans' (2015) newly published and in most regards invaluable *Actor Training Reader*, inviting them to search the index for references to speech (as distinct from the still marginalized category of voice). This was my visual aid deployed in a bid to persuade participants that our contemporary intellectual/artistic community has devoted itself to an ideal of the 'physical' at the expense of one of the most crucial of the body's activities. I also used a more conventional visual aid, to which I could impart less physical energy – a Power-Point of Meisner's dichotomy: 'An ounce of behavior is worth a pound of words.' In our technologized culture, speech as the meeting point between behaviour and words has somehow gone AWOL.

At the time of writing, I am working on French theatre, and vivid in my mind is the fate of the great actor Mondory, who starred in Corneille's *Le Cid* in 1637 and specialized in big emotions rather than characterisation (Merlin 2008). At the climax of another tragic role a few months later, his physical exertion was such that he suffered a left-hemisphere stroke on stage which disabled both his voice and his right arm. He tried to make a comeback but only found himself able to perform in the intimacy of a court theatre. The fate of Mondory illustrates the interconnectedness of emotion, voice and gesture. We are hardwired to gesture when we speak because making words involves, in our imaginations and mus-cular systems, moulding objects – which of course helps resolve the great evo-lutionary conundrum: did humans become human through speech or through using tools? In stress-based languages like English, our bodies demand not only to create shapes but also to beat time because tempo-rhythms (as Stanislavski understood so well) are inseparable from emotional expression. If I were reading this text aloud to you, I would no longer be making my words afresh, and gesture would largely disappear – whence the tedium of so many academic conferences geared towards publication. One of the key things we can learn from the classical tradition is the interconnection between the making of language and the perfor-mance of language.

To illustrate my proposition about language as substance, I will put before you an extended quotation from the works of the playwright and sometime actor Ben Jonson (1572–1637). The text is from his commonplace book, and translates or paraphrases a passage he particularly liked in the work of the Spanish scholar, Juan Luis Vives (1493–1540) who amongst other things, tutored Princess Mary of England. Vives argued that speech 'springs out of the most retired and inmost parts of us,' and so we should analyse it in exactly the same terms as we analyse the body, in terms of its size, shape and surface features, and the substance of which it is made. (Human juice in Vives' (2002) physiological model is veinous blood that resembles the sap of a tree.)

> The next thing to the stature, is the figure and feature in Language: that is, whether it be round, and streight, which consists of short and succinct *Periods*, numerous, and polish'd, or square and firme; which is to have equall and strong parts, every where answerable, and weighed. The third is the skinne, and coat, which rests in the well-joyning, cementing, and coagmentation of words; when as it is smooth, gentle, and sweet; like a Table, upon which you may runne your finger without rubs, and your nayle cannot find a joynt; not horrid, rough, wrinckled, gaping, or chapt: After these the flesh, blood, and bones come in question. Wee say it is a fleshy style, when there is much *Periphrases*, and circuit of words; and when with more then enough, it growes fat and corpulent; *Arvina orationis*, full of suet and tallow. It hath blood, and juyce, when the words are proper and apt, their sound sweet, and the *Phrase* neat and pick'd. *Oratio uncta, & benè pasta.* But where there is Redundancy, both the blood and juyce are faulty, and vitious. *Redundat sanguine, quâ multô plus dicit, quàm necesse est.* Juyce in Language is some what lesse then blood; for if the words be but becomming, and signifying, and the sense gentle, there is Juyce: but where that wanteth, the Language is thinne, flagging, poore, starv'd; scarce covering the bone; and shewes like stones in a sack. Some men to avoid Redundancy, runne into that; and while they strive to have no ill blood, or Juyce, they loose their good. There be some styles againe, that have not lesse blood, but lesse flesh, and corpulence. These are bony, and sinnewy: *Ossa habent, et nervos.*
>
> (Jonson 2012: 567–70)

It may test your patience to read this long citation in old spelling. We live accelerated lives in the 21st century that pressure us to reach for the key point rather than savour the quality of prose. The editorial feedback that I and my fellow contributors to this volume receive on our drafts will inevitably concentrate on the structuring of our argument, and its relevance to the theme of temporality, and because times have changed, will probably not comment on whether our style is bloodless or corpulent, smooth or lumpy.

I have preserved the old spelling in my citation, and of course I could have modernized it in order to make the 'meaning' clearer, your reading quicker and more efficient. However, … if you feel able to linger on the italicized Latin, you can sense how Jonson is engaged in a conversation, hearing another voice speaking to him from a century earlier. If you can afford the time, notice how the capitalisation of 'Table' encourages you to picture the object, while the old spelling of 'runne' draws out the monosyllable so your muscular impulses can participate in the act of running a finger along polished wood, and likewise to hit the final consonant of 'nayle' is to experience the precision of Jonson's search for a crack in the joinery. Or take the punctuation – a colon after 'chapt,' a full stop after 'question.' Today we would punctuate the other way round, but Jonson punctuates for time not syntax. The reader/speaker needs to pause after 'question' so the listener (maybe the same person) can digest and place in short-term memory the three categories of flesh, blood and bone that will be treated in sequence. Or consider the emotional force of the semicolons before and after 'scarce covering the bone' – signals to pause longer than required for a comma so the image of horror can be felt. Jonson's language invites us to feel what he is saying as much as to understand, because thinking cannot ultimately be separated from feeling.

The inseparability of emotion and cognition is today widely acknowledged, even if the implications are ignored, and creative arts departments for ever have to struggle against institutional structures that look to an ideal of pure rationality. To find the way forward, it may be helpful to look backwards to a time when an educational system based on rhetoric put a far higher premium on performance. The rhetorical tradition understood that the art of timing was central to performance, because texts were never just static objects but always seen as a form of vocal score. The problem to my mind started in the Enlightenment, when words were taken as the vehicles of essential meanings, and plays taken to be vehicles for a moral point made by the playwright rather than a form of social encounter. And people forgot that performance was also a means to develop a set of common rhythms with an audience, one of the fundamental devices for human bonding.

Is the idea of renewing the rhetorical system of actor training merely a flight of my academic fancy? Adonis Galeos is a former student of mine, an actor and dramaturg deeply read in the rhetorical literature of early modern England, and he has made rhetoric the foundation of a training programme in a private drama school in Athens. I have not witnessed the work so I will only quote a snippet from his course outline:

> This intensive module explores the potentials generated by the application of rhetorical theory on contemporary actor training … Scholars and prac-titioners throughout the ages have viewed rhetoric as a way of knowing, as a way of being, and as a way of presenting oneself (double consciousness) … The course will be structured around three educational cycles: Rhetorical figures and tropes as the foundation for the embodiment of the part, mem-orization as a trigger for imagination, inventing a structure as a means to influence the emotions of the audience.[2]

I unpack this as follows: (1) The starting point lies not in the fixing of character but in developing the creative gap between the orator/actor and the speech/role, finding the role in patterns of speech and as it were taking Brecht into Derrida. (2) Memorising words is not the chore which it is taken to be in a world of instant access to digitized knowledge, but a means of perceiving shape and pattern, in and beyond language. (3) The actor is an active maker of texts and situations; the focus of his or her training is not upon transformation but upon the quality of interaction with a specific audience. The rhetorical system is of course as open to interpretation as the Stanislavskian system, and this is merely one individual's approach.

The point of my short contribution to this volume is simply to insist that looking backwards may be the best way to look forwards. The premodern world points us towards a long-standing and coherent tradition of training which starts from the premise that live theatre is first and foremost a social interaction, a means by which one or more actors work on the emotions of an audience. How we access the principles of that tradition is the focus of my current research, and beyond my scope to address here. As a historian, what I want to emphasize by way of conclusion is that we live within the flux of history. Yet the accelerated pace of modern living causes memories to become shorter and shorter. Anyone involved in training draws upon methods and exercises that have worked for them in the past in order to prepare actors for an unknown future when the world will have changed. We are all products of history, but like to think that our recipes for artistic success are somehow timeless.

Notes

1 TaPRA is the UK-based Theatre and Performance Research Association.
2 Unpublished course materials prepared for the Delos Drama School, Athens, 2013.

References

Evans, M. (ed.) (2015) *The Actor Training Reader*, London: Routledge.
Jonson, B. (2012) 'Timber – or, Discoveriesï, ed. Lorna Hutson,' in Bevington, D.M., Butler, M. and Donaldson, I. (eds) *The Cambridge Edition of the Works of Ben Jonson, Vol. VII*, Cambridge: Cambridge University Press.
Merlin, H. (2008) 'Effets de voix, effets de scène: Mondory entre le *Cid* et la *Marianne*,' in Rosenthal, O. (ed.) *À Haute voix. diction et prononciation aux XVIe et XVIIe siècles*, Paris: Klincksieck, 155–76.
Quintilian, M.F. (2001) *The Orator's Education*, ed. and transl. D. Russell, Cambridge, MA: Harvard University Press.
Roach, J.R. (1985) *The Player's Passion: Studies in the Science of Acting*, Ann Arbor: University of Michigan Press.
Vives, J.L. (2002) *De Ratione Dicendi*, ed. E. Mattioli, Napoli: La città del sole.

5

TIME IN NOH THEATRE PERFORMANCE AND TRAINING

Conversations with Udaka Tatsushige

Diego Pellecchia

Learning about noh theatre, a traditional Japanese performing art combining poetry, music and movement, one often encounters keywords such as *jo-ha-kyū*, *ma* or *ichi-go ichi-e*, all of which are expressions of time. For noh performers, 'timeliness', or the ability to catch the 'right time,' does not only refer to musical ability, but also to 'readiness' to act effectively whenever required with little or no notice. Despite training as main role specialists, *shite* actors have limited chances to perform such roles, hence it is essential for them to be ready to catch these occasions, which may only occur once in their lifetime. To prepare for such events, noh actors begin training at a very young age and dedicate their lives to polishing their art. In this article, we would like to introduce notions of time in the training of a *shite* actor, and place them within the larger context of a noh play production.

Seasons of noh

Many forms of Japanese contemporary and traditional culture, from language to art, from fashion to cuisine, abound with references to nature and its cyclical transformations. Since the beginning of Japanese literature in the 8th century, plants, animals or other natural phenomena became literary *tropes*, representing different seasons. For example, the bush warbler signifies spring, while the moon is associated with autumn. Such concepts have been codified in poetic anthologies, establishing what Shirane Haruo called 'secondary nature' (Shirane 2012, 4), that is, culturally construed conceptions of nature which became models for artistic production and appreciation.

Noh theatre, emerging in the 14th century as the confluence of previously existing genres, is part of the same tradition. The current noh repertoire comprises of about 200 plays, most of which are classified according to the season they represent (Okazaki 1985). For example, Kiyomizu Temple surrounded by cherry blossoms is the background of *Tamura*, a spring play; the spirit of the Water Iris is the protagonist of *Kakitsubata*, a summer play; *Momijigari* is set against the backdrop of Arashiyama's famous maple red foliage in autumn; in *Yuki*, a winter play, the protagonist is the spirit of the snow.

The everyday life of the noh community of performers and audience is punctuated by the rhythm of the noh calendar, based on seasonal rituality rather than case-by-case contracts with producers. In early January, attending the celebratory performance *Okina*, reminiscent of ancient agricultural rites in which benevolent deities bestow blessings on the land, is part of the New Year rituals. From January until December, regular performances at specialized playhouses take place monthly, though noh is also regularly staged at temples and shrines during festivals. Plays to be staged are carefully chosen in accordance with the season, to the extent that they may be considered as 'time-specific performances,' blending the natural conditions experienced offstage with the fictional nature of the onstage narrative. In some cases, plays are purposely chosen in contrast with the season during which they are staged. For example, a winter play may be performed in the summer to bring the audience relief from the heat.

Noh times

The time of performance cross-fades with that of everyday life. Upon entering a modern noh playhouse to watch a play, one notices that the bare stage is in plain sight. The lights are only slightly dimmed and, while the spectators are still looking at the program or checking their mobile phones, the musicians and chorus quietly enter the stage, unannounced.

A noh performance follows a tripartite, cyclical structure called *jo-ha-kyū* (lit. 'begin-break-fast'), which can be observed at a microscopic level, as in the movement of the arm of a dancer, and at a macroscopic level, as in the longer timespan of a performance day. The introductory section of a play (*jo*) is accompanied by a slow-tempo introductory music in which the musicians fill the long pauses between beats with protracted shouts emphasizing the *ma*, a term used to describe spatiotemporal 'in-betweenness.' When the tempo is particularly low, such pauses last up to several seconds, stretching beyond the human sense of rhythm. Drum patterns are played in loops, and their slowness often generates different effects on the spectators: some of them try to resist the feeling of uneasiness caused by the unbearable heaviness of *jo*, so distant from the faster pace of life experienced in offstage, everyday life. Others surrender to the hypnosis of the drummers, perhaps drifting into a dreamlike state.

In noh, narrative time is flexible: it can be condensed, expanded or reversed (Komparu 1983: 70–8). For example, in the dramaturgical format called *mugen-noh*, 'noh of dream and illusion,' the *shite*, a deity, ghost or a spirit appears in disguise in front the *waki*, a common man. In the second half of the play, the *shite* reappears in his or her real shape and enacts past events, for example, in the case of a ghost warrior, his tragic death in battle. Here, two time dimensions overlap: the past from which the *shite* emerges, and the present which he inhabits together with the *waki*. This narrative type is rooted in Buddhist notions of impermanence, emphasising the fleeting nature of earthly existence, and rebirth, by which human actions have consequences that lead to future existences after death, in an endless cycle.

The plot develops during the *ha* phase, rhythmically faster, but longer than *jo*. Finally, the play closes with *kyū*, which is shorter and lighter, and may be felt as a liberation from the oppressive weight accumulated in the previous sections. As the performance comes to an end, the performers slowly exit the stage, without coming back to receive the applause. The stage reverts to its bare condition, as it was before the performance began. The cycle is completed.

The time of production

One of the most peculiar features of noh is that its performances are one-off events, never repeated on consecutive days. This convention follows an aesthetic-ethical principle that can be described with the expression *ichi-go ichi-e*, 'one time, one meeting,' according to which life events such as a meeting of people should be treasured as unique happenings. Likewise, noh performances may be seen as nodal points in which the separate lifelines of its participants – both performers and spectators – intertwine for a limited and unrepeatable period. Theatre scholar Peggy Phelan notably pointed out that 'performance occurs over a time which will not be repeated. It can be performed again, but this repetition itself marks it as "different"' (Phelan 1993: 146). Japanese traditional arts took the idea of performance as an ontologically irreproducible act, codified it and made it one of their supreme aesthetic-ethical principles.

As there is only one staging of a noh play, so there is only one rehearsal – an abridged run-through without costumes and masks – taking place just a few days before the actual performance. This is the only chance for the actors and musicians to check what they have until that moment studied individually. This process is technically possible because of two basic reasons. First, all aspects of the performance text are codified into a canon shared across all performers. Second, noh performers specialize only in one role (*shite*, *waki*, *kyōgen* or one of the four instruments), and although they train separately, most of them are involved exclusively in noh productions. Therefore, as the training of all performers is based on the same material, rehearsing with the rest of the cast is not necessary as long as training is carried out successfully. In this sense, a noh performance resembles a jazz session, in which rehearsing would deprive the performance of the 'genuineness' originating from the irreproducible live event. This view of performance expresses an ethical quality of 'truthfulness' despite the artificiality of the theatrical production. Noh dramaturgy and audio-visual aesthetics blatantly lack realism: it aims at being 'natural' without being 'naturalist,' a paradox is encapsulated in the expression *musakui no sakui*, 'planned spontaneity'.

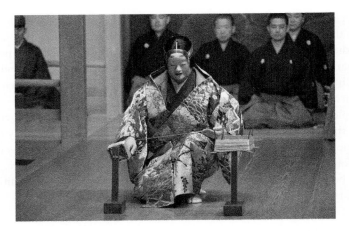

FIGURE 5.1 Udaka Tatsushige in the noh *Kurozuka*, 25 September 2016, Kongō Noh Theatre, Kyoto. In *Kurozuka*, a woman (actually a monster in disguise) laments the long seasons spent alone in the mountains, spinning threads for a living. The gesture of spinning is also a metaphor of the cycle of rebirth. Photo: Fabio Massimo Fioravanti.

Training seasons

Shite actors can perform in three capacities: as *shite* (main role) or *tsure* (secondary role), as a chorus member, or as a stage assistant. While *shite* are often hired to perform as chorus members or stage assistants, for most of these actors, performing as *shite* is the supreme expression of their art, an event occurring only a few times in a year. It follows that a certain performance may be the first and last time an actor can take the *shite* role in a certain play of the repertoire. However, as seasonality implies not only change but also cyclical recurrence, actors may perform the *shite* role of a play multiple times in their lives, albeit with a different cast and often with the addition of performance variations. In any case, given the limited chances to perform, *shite* actors need to train intensively to be ready to catch what may be the only chance to perform the main role in a play. Long study periods are the prelude to one single performance event.

The training of a *shite* actor can be roughly subdivided into two main phases. The first is a 'formative phase': a period of apprenticeship beginning when actors are about three years old and usually continuing until their mid-twenties, when they become fully independent performers. The second is a 'perfecting phase,' which begins with their professional independence, and continues until the end of their artistic career, often coinciding with physical incapability to perform, or death.

During the 'formative phase,' actors learn the basics of their art: how to sing, act and dance. Actors should also study most if not all four instruments of the noh orchestra: flute, shoulder drum, hip drum and stick drum. *Shite* actors also learn all aspects of the backstage work: how to prepare, fold and store costumes, and how to dress other actors. They also learn how to operate the *agemaku* pull-up curtain at the end of the *hashigakari* bridgeway connecting the backstage with the main stage, as well as how to prepare and handle stage properties. As a result, of all noh performers, *shite* actors have the most comprehensive knowledge of performance: a well-trained *shite* is aware all aspects of performance – onstage, backstage, offstage – as it happens.

Initially, the training of children takes place in one-to-one sessions in which the teacher demonstrates the model and the student tries to imitate it as closely as possible. During the first years of their formation, children appear on stage as *kokata* (child roles) along with adult actors. Later, they are taught simple *shimai*, dance-chant excerpts from longer plays performed without costumes and masks. With puberty, children undergo voice change: it is during this time that they start studying music and learning the basics of dance. Children around this age may also perform *shite* main roles in full performances, although without a mask.

During their youth, most actors train either as 'live-in' or 'commuting' apprentices of the *iemoto*, the grand master of a noh school. The timing of this phase varies, but it generally occurs when the actor is between 15 and 25 years old.[1] During this phase, trainees learn how to take care of stage, costumes, masks, properties, but are also asked to perform everyday chores such as cleaning, shopping or driving. Living together with the teacher provides students with maximum exposure both to the artistic and to the everyday life of a full professional.

However, during this period, one-to-one lessons with the teacher are sparse. The student is supposed to have acquired sufficient tools to study independently. Most of the student's training time is spent practising what they learnt in the previous class, and getting ready for the next meeting. Lessons are chances to check what the actor has studied alone and to receive corrections and instructions for the following piece of study, and they may be as short as just a few minutes. Like performances, lessons are *ichi-go ichi-e* moments, to be treasured as unique and unrepeatable.

In Japanese traditional arts, training is called *keiko*, or 'to ponder on past things.' Rather than a creative endeavour, *keiko* is a process of internalisation of pre-existent knowledge. In the case of noh, this knowledge is the result of over six centuries of stratification, mutation and transmission. Noh gained popularity during the early Muromachi period (1336–1573) also thanks to the endeavours of Kan'ami Kiyotsugu and his son Zeami Motokiyo, who were playwrights, actors and troupe managers. Zeami, whose playwriting style defined a dramaturgical standard, left a rich corpus of writings in which he reflects not only on various aspects of composition and performance, but also on training. In his treatise *Fūshikaden* (in Thomas Hare's translation, 'Transmitting the Flower Through Effects and Attitudes'), Zeami describes training across seven stages of life, from infancy to maturity, and beyond (Zeami 2008: 26–31). Particularly concerned with the transmission of his art to posterity, Zeami advised: 'study the old, then, and make certain that you do not neglect tradition even while appreciating the new'

(Zeami 2008: 26). Even today, as the one-to-one, direct mode of transmission between master and pupil emphasizes lineage, trainees grow an awareness of their position on the noh timeline in relation to their ancestors and to their future role within the noh world.

During the latter part of the 'formative phase,' actors spend a great amount of time in the solitary activity of memorising chants for a core group of some one hundred frequently performed plays. Actors often carry miniature-size chant books to continue their study during idle times such as train commutes, or between other lessons. At the end of this training phase, actors are ready to perform such plays with little or no notice.

As actors complete their formation, they enter the 'perfecting phase,' in which they build on what they have learned during the first phase in a sort of 'augmentative repetition.' During this period, they polish their execution of core plays while they learn less-performed plays and new variants. While training in the formative phase is mostly based on imitation of teachers and seniors, during the perfecting phase, actors develop their own individual style. Noh is *over-trained*, a condition made possible by exclusive specialisation, which is in turn necessary to acquire mastery of the many facets of the profession. Actors need to interiorize a large repertoire of plays and being able to perform them with short or no notice. However, noh is also *under-rehearsed*, as over-training would result in mechanical repetition leading to a predictable performance. Actors accumulate solitary training hours and release the result of their work only on the one performance day.

From the point of view of the audience, the training of an actor may be compared to the *ma*, the interval between beats in noh music. Just as the prolonged shouts of the musicians create an expectation for the beat which will come at their end, the absence from the stage between performances generates expectation for the progress of the actor the next time he or she will appear in front of the audience.

Time in performance

As already indicated, actors have only a few chances to perform the *shite* role, for which they have trained since their infancy. What kind of awareness of time (within this unrepeatable event) do actors have on stage? Since in the staging of a noh play all elements are fixed, if the actor is prepared, then the only necessary thing to do is to recall a scenic text stored in the memory during innumerable repetitions and to follow the flow of a pre-established plan. However, this plan is not always a one-way road, and an actor must consider the different possible consequences that a certain movement may cause. In *Theatre and Time*, David Wiles points out how 'Stanislavski's method is future oriented: it asks the actor to focus on the task ahead, and the audience to wait in anticipation' (Wiles 2014: 51). Although noh does not request performers to analyse the psychology of characters to find motivations for their actions, it necessarily urges the actor to be aware of the task ahead to play 'on time' both in musical and choreutic terms. For example, actor Fukuō Shigejūrō describes how, in the play *Chōryō*, the *waki* needs to recover a shoe thrown by the *shite* (Fukuō and Kamimura 2017: 2). The trajectory of the thrown shoe is unpredictable, yet the *waki* must be ready to recover the shoe regardless of where it lands, which may be different parts of the stage or even off the stage. While the *waki* must consider how to act in spontaneous response to the events on stage, he will be able to perform the movement convincingly only if he has experienced all possible shoe landings during training.[2] Thorough knowledge of performance, and an extensive training that considers different possible scenarios, enables the actor to catch the one chance to perform on stage successfully. To this extent, the training of the noh actor resembles that of an athlete: they both spend long hours not only perfecting movements and rehearsing routines, but also considering various ways the performance will unfold on the performance day.

Noh performances do not occur in a time dimension disjointed from that of the audience: as it is not possible to put life on pause, a noh performance cannot be interrupted. *Shite* assistants, sitting on stage throughout the performance, are supposed to take on the *shite*'s role in case of an accident, as noh performance should not be interrupted. On 1 June 2016, during the performance of Zeami's masterpiece *Kakitsubata* ('The Water Iris') at Heian Shrine in Kyoto, the flute player suffered a heart attack and passed away on stage. While stage assistants and paramedics were assisting him, another flutist took his place and continued to perform until the end of the play. Time did not stop, instead tradition, in its literal sense, happened before the eyes of its participants.

Notes

1 Recently, even those born into families of professionals tend to follow a regular study course. As a consequence, they may become live-in apprentices after university graduation.
2 The male pronoun is used here as all waki actors are men.

References

Fukuō, S. and Kamimura, T. (2017, 1st Sept.) 'Nō No Shōrai Wo Kangaeru (Considering the Future of Noh),' *Nōgaku Times.*

Komparu, K. (1983) *The Noh Theater: Principles and Perspectives*, New York: Weatherhill/ Tankosha.

Okazaki, T. (1985) 'Yōkyoku to Kisetsu (Noh Plays and the Seasons),' *Komazawa University Tandaikokubun*, 15(March): 1–17.

Phelan, P. (1993) *Unmarked: The Politics of Performance*, London and New York: Routledge.

Shirane, H. (2012) *Japan and the Culture of the Four Seasons: Nature, Literature, and the Arts*, New York: Columbia University Press.

Wiles, D. (2014) *Theatre & Time*, Basingstoke: Palgrave.

Zeami, M. (2008) *Performance Notes*, trans. T. Hare, New York: Columbia University Press.

6

A MATERIALIST FEMINIST PERSPECTIVE ON TIME IN ACTOR TRAINING

The commodity of illusion

Evi Stamatiou

During a module feedback session with UK conservatoire trainees in November 2014, I asked the class: 'Did you find it valuable that during the training process we considered the inequalities that women face in the acting field?' A female trainee responded: 'No. I would rather concentrate on my acting now and not worry about the future.' Writing from the perspective of an actor and actor-trainer, I aim to raise awareness about the fact that temporality in actor-training, considered in socio-economic terms, is different for women. I will explore temporality using Gary Becker's concept of 'human capital' (2009: 12) which enables me to analyse the risks of a woman's time investment in actor training for her future socio-economic prospects. A socio-economic notion of time emerges from this analysis: time as a commodity of illusion.

Using a materialist feminist approach, I critically analyse the use of time in actor-training. I use quantitative data, such as gender-related statistics relating to employment and training from Purple Seven[1] and the Universities and Colleges Admissions Service (UCAS). I also use qualitative data, such as reports about undergraduate students' rights under consumer law from the Competition & Markets Authority (CMA); key findings about employability from the Higher Education Academy (HEA); actor-training practices, such as classical text-based training and cross-casting; and anonymized participants' testimonies. This analysis highlights the fact that it is paradoxical for a person to invest their time in actor training if their gender, race, ability and other embodied characteristics mean that their commodified body is a less desirable product. It contributes to contemporary debates about the 'political turn' in actor training – Maria Kapsali writes that the interrogation of the political nature of actor-training 'has now acquired an urgent, pragmatic and ethical dimension' (2014a: 104) – and raises awareness about the ethical implications for actor-training institutions which do not directly address the challenging employability perspectives for women.

Women's experience of time in training has been affected by material changes in the UK during the last decade: arts funding has been cut, traditional conservatoires have been increasingly merged with universities and university fees have been increased. Following the 2008 economic crisis, the Arts Council of England and the British Film Institute lost 15% of their funding (HM Treasury 2010: 65), which immediately affected the acting field. Local government spending on arts and culture between 2010 and 2015 has also declined by 16.6% (Harvey 2015: 9), which indicates that job opportunities for actors in the UK in the last decade have declined by more than 15%. These significant cuts in funding are likely to continue (Harvey 2015: 10) and therefore employability of actors will probably deteriorate.

Another factor that affected employability in the acting sector is the merging or association of conservatoires and universities. As a result of this 'the courses studied at these drama schools have become three-year degrees rather than diplomas' (Prior 2012: 79), which indicates that women spend 33% more time in training than before. Also, there has been 'an increased number of places available to students' (ibid.), which further affects the already saturated market of the acting field. This gloomy picture gets worse with the introduction and the increase of university fees: a £1,000 per year fee was introduced in 1998, which was raised to £3,000 in 2004 and £9,000 in 2009. Such changes have affected both the trainee's experience of time in training in relation to economic returns from acting jobs and also their increased expectations from actor-training institutions. As CMA suggests, since 2015, the trainee/institution relationship is a consumer/provider relationship, 'together with the existence of a supportive learning and pastoral environment within an academic community' (CMA 2015b: 3). The fact that the broader interest in the politics of actor-training in the 2000s (Kapsali 2014a: 103) began at the same time that the trainee became an economic agent, invites us to consider the trainee's socio-economic agency in relation to actor training as socio-economic temporality.

The materialities of the present

Women trainees' material experience of the present is influenced by educational institutions' structures and goals. Alison Hodge suggests that traditionally, the ultimate goal of actor-training institutions, which is also true for most contemporary actor-training institutions, is 'to prepare the actor for work' (2000: 2). This suggests that trainees' time in the institutions was always projected into the future. My materialist feminist lens focuses on how the preparation of the actor for work and its relation to the economy affects how the female trainee is projected into the future.

The economic changes of the last decade, which have been driven by a neo-liberal agenda that seeks the privatization of higher education, are primarily institutional changes that affect the present and future experience of the female trainee. The trainee's relationship with the actor-training institution depends on their 'provider-consumer' contract. After being accepted on a course, she signs a 'consumer contract' with the 'business'/educational institution (CMA 2015b: 17). This works for both parties: a trainee needs to fulfil her economic obligations to the institution and the institution needs to acknowledge the duties and responsibilities of their side of the contract. Higher education has increasingly adopted managerial models of organization from industry and commerce (Ridout 2014: 77), which have established the idea that actor-training institutions should consider professionalization not only as production of 'professional actors' but also as providers of skills that aim for sustainable professional careers for the trainees, which is determined by the economic returns on jobs that are a result of the specific degree. Such changes lead actor training to see the actor's work not only as 'an aesthetic, artistic and affective dimension [...] [but as] a form of labour with a monetary and cultural value and, as such, subject to a wider set of political and economic transactions' (Kapsali 2014a: 106). The structure and nature of actor-training institutions and the socio-economic temporality of training urges us to consider time in training as a form of investment with a monetary and social value. As such, it is subject to a wider set of socio-economic transactions.

Considering the woman trainee as a socio-economic agent brings attention to her monetary investment in training and how it generates money in the future through acting jobs. The CMA considers it a necessity that Higher Education students should be protected by consumer rights law because enrolment on a course is often 'a 'one-off' decision involving the investment of a significant amount of time and money' (CMA 2015b: 3). Women's time in training represents investment that they expect to get them a return in terms of acting jobs in the future. They acquire knowledge about how to act and how to get an acting job. Thinking about the trainee's time as 'invested,' 'spent' or 'wasted' under such capitalist terms invites the economist Becker's concept of human capital.

Human capital is an individual's investment in their education, or other activities such as medical care, migration or searching for information about prices and income. In most cases, it results in a higher income (Becker 2009: 12). To calculate human capital during actor-training, it is necessary to consider both direct expenses, such as the tuition fees, and indirect expenses, for example, if women were not in training they might be working and earning money. Becker, who applies the term to education, has been criticized for referring only to monetary value.[2] If actor-training institutions consider themselves service-providing businesses and their trainees consumers, this affects the number of trainees they recruit and train: the more students they train, the bigger their profit. However, this produces more qualified actors and further saturates the acting market, which means that getting a job is getting more difficult whereas getting a degree is getting easier. To tackle the highly competitive market, actor-training institutions insist on promoting trainees' employability and transferrable skills. Therefore, human capital is an appropriate term. This form of capital is called 'human' and not 'physical' or 'financial' because knowledge or skills cannot be separated from the person, unlike physical or financial assets (Becker 2009: 16). The trainee invests in her own acting knowledge, from which she cannot be separated. The investment is deposited as she goes through training and acquires knowledge, and her earnings are expected to rise as she begins to work in the economy.

On the other hand, every investment has an associated risk, and the rates of return on education, in monetary terms, and not the same for all individuals.[3] Becker suggests that an individual's incentive to invest in education is determined by how they perceive the job market: they see which careers will give them higher-earning jobs and they invest in the relevant education (2009: 9). This is important, because it highlights the paradox that women trainees invest in actor training in higher numbers than their male counterparts, even though they are aware of how much more challenging the acting profession is for them. Women are the majority of trainees across conservatoire and university actor-training courses.[4] A 66% rise in the acceptance of women applicants in 2016 mirrors a general rise in acceptances in higher education, and its main aim is to generate more profit from trainees' fees for actor-training institutions (UCAS 2016a). According to 'UCAS conservatoires end of cycle report 2015,' following a 17% rise in applications and acceptances from the previous year, the total application numbers indicate that women are 60% more are likely to apply and be accepted (2016b: 22). The number of women applying is even higher for drama-specific courses (UCAS 2015: 3). This indicates that female trainees' incentive to invest in education is not immediately related to the job market.

Applicants who fail to get on to a conservatoire actor-training course often reapply to conservatoires or enrol on university drama courses: data demonstrates that 67.4% of women who applied through UCAS conservatoires for drama-specific courses also applied for drama courses through UCAS undergraduate (UCAS 2016c: 26). Again, most applicants and acceptances on these courses are women (ibid: 33), with acceptances for drama courses in 2016 reaching 2,385 men and 5,545 women (UCAS 2016b: W4).[5] Even though drama-specific university students do not necessarily aim for the acting field, many of them often do and the recent turn of universities towards professionalization in order to enhance the employability prospects of their students, adds to the overall number of women who compete for acting jobs.

As UCAS's data demonstrates, women train on courses in which the majority of other trainees are women. The paradox is that this not only does not improve women's experience, but on the contrary makes the whole training process more stressful and unequal, especially with regard to text-based work. Female trainees face more competition during training, because there are fewer parts for women in classical and contemporary writing.[6] For example, when I trained actors on a UK undergraduate conservatoire course in 2014, the group consisted of eleven women and seven men. The module lasted 12 weeks from October to December and included the staging of two works: Shakespeare's *Richard III* and Joseph Stein, Sheldon Harnick and Jerry Bock's musical *Fiddler on the Roof.*

In both works, the main character and most of the supporting characters are men. There were few supporting roles for the women.

Rehearsal and stage time in conservatoire productions is typically distributed according to the roles in the full production. The male characters in the works had more stage time, and it was divided among the seven men, whereas the female characters had less stage time, and it was divided among the eleven women. Therefore, although the women paid the same fees, they got less rehearsal and stage time during training, leaving them with a time-quantity disadvantage. However, there was also a time-quality disadvantage: the main characters, Richard in *Richard III* and Tevye in *Fiddler on the Roof*, are written with more depth than the female supporting characters. Consequently, the women had fewer opportunities to develop their acting skills. Therefore, the women in the cohort were disadvantaged in their overall experience of time in actor training.

The experience of these female trainees is common. The Bechdel Test[7] highlights that most texts give more time to men, and that women's parts are generally less important. Gender bias is acknowledged to be a problem on stage, especially in classical works, such as *Richard III* and *Fiddler on the Roof*, which are often used in text-based training within conservatoires. Therefore, the texts used in actor-training disadvantage women's socio-economic temporality and career prospects: women are given less time, both quantitatively and qualitatively, to develop their acting skills, even though they should be better prepared than men for a more challenging future. This inequality of experience and opportunity is not only an ethical issue but also something that higher education institutions are required to address, as indicated in the Quality Code for Drama, Dance and Performance from the Quality Assurance Agency for Higher Education (2015: 3). Many actor trainers understand this, which is why works like Federico García Lorca's *The House of Bernarda Alba* and the musical *Sister Act* are popular in conservatoires' repertoires. However, because contemporary UK actor-training does not officially address the gender inequality of time, most women are likely to be subjected to repertoires like the one I described above.

I discussed the inequalities women face in the acting field with the class I trained because I wanted everyone to make a shared decision about how the parts would be distributed among the trainees, and therefore how rehearsal and stage time would be allocated. For example, I suggested using cross-casting, which is a useful casting device that solves the challenge of having a majority of women trainees and a repertoire that limits casting opportunities for women. The women in the class did not want to spend six weeks rehearsing and performing the role of the main character, Tevye, because they felt that taking on a part that they would never perform in the industry was a waste of time. They said they would rather train as Tevye's daughters – although the characters have smaller parts, are limited in depth and are always discussing marriage – because that is how they assumed that they would be cast after graduation. Their acceptance of this time inequality in training foresees a future of surrendering to the broader inequalities of the acting industry.

The materialities of the future

Many women invest their time in actor-training, even though the current situation in the acting industry shows that future prospects for women are disappointing. Kapsali observes that even when employed, 'performing arts graduates will most likely be engaged in an industry that shows alarming signs of deregulation, low remuneration and gruelling working conditions' (2014a: 104). The unemployment rate for actors reached 92%, and it has been suggested that the other 8% is the same people constantly in employment (Simkins 2009). Since 2009, the situation has worsened, as the cuts to arts funding have led to a situation in which 'more than half of actors are under [the] poverty line' (Vincent 2014). Jen Harvie describes the 'real' actors' jobs in the West:

> To remain available to compete whenever a suitable audition comes up, so-called resting actors between acting contracts generally do anything but rest, needing to take jobs, but jobs that are flexible so that they can be dropped at short notice. The actor's typical 'resting' jobs – office temp, cleaner, waiter – are indeed comparatively flexible, but also therefore comparatively insecure and ill-paid.
>
> *(2009: 39)*

The acting profession, as labour that brings in money, is not only precarious but hardly 'real' for most actors, especially if they have the worst characteristic of all in regards to succeeding as an actor – in other words, if they are a woman (Willmott 2015). Data from Purple Seven reveals that, amongst employed actors, only 39% are women (2015). Therefore, women are more likely to spend most of their time looking for acting jobs while working in other positions. Given that looking for jobs and enduring temping is a fundamental part of an actor's future career, especially if she is a woman, actor-training institutions that promise 'employability' should arguably develop a curriculum that devotes at least 50% of the time to preparing actors for job-searching.

Conservatoire training has traditionally linked job-searching with auditions, which are usually a result of a talent agent putting an actor forward for a specific role. Actors are not typically encouraged to be proactive: traditional conservatoire training assumes that actors must wait to be employed by casting agents and directors. The first step for the trainee after graduation is to find a talent agent, but the 'best actors often don't sign with an agent, because they are young, white, brown-haired women who are over-represented in the industry, and have fewer opportunities for work' (Alexander in Kapsali 2014b: 223). If women cannot get talent agents, they are less likely to get well-paid acting jobs.

The fact that most trainee actors in the UK are women is at odds with the realities of the acting profession for women. This might lead us to think that female trainee actors are less competent in judging profitable investments or more willing to take on risk, but I would suggest another possibility: they consciously buy the systemic illusion for a 'hopeful future.'[8] Actor-training institutions compete in the relevant education market and their desire to attract applicants often leads to the promise of career prospects that are unrealistic (Tibby 2012: 6), and this further sustains the illusion. To the extent that an employability agenda attempts to unrealistically relate training time to future employability, the female trainee's time in actor-training is experienced as an illusionary investment in human capital.

Frank Camilleri writes that actor training in the contemporary West is a commodity sold by institutions and bought by students (2009: 34), which echoes Brecht's and Anderson's description of knowledge as a commodity that is acquired to be resold (1961: 21). However, the material conditions of the acting profession indicate that the acting knowledge is less likely to be resold, which means that female trainees buy a 'commodity of illusion.' Because female trainees consciously buy the 'commodity of illusion' within a systemic neo-liberal agenda of a 'hopeful future,' contemporary actor-training institutions are morally responsible for taking action: acting knowledge is not a waste of time and money after the trainee has managed to get a job, which indicates that 'getting acting jobs skills' needs to be prioritized over 'acting skills.'

Most of the trainee's time in conservatoire actor-training is spent on 'acting skills,' which are achieved primarily by putting on productions, especially in the last year of training. Although acting in a public production gives the actor more experience, the institutions' primary aims are to use such productions in order to attract talent agents (Prior 2012: 79), which is a central point of attraction for applicants. Given that talent agents make a decision after seeing a trainee only once, repeated public productions seem like a waste of time and money. Public productions are aimed at only one employability option – talent agents – and trainees do not develop other skills they need to get a job. Although conservatoires boast about their achievements in getting talent agents for trainees, not all trainees get an agent and, even if they do, it does not guarantee work (Prior 2012: 80).

Actor training courses tackle the need for getting acting job skills with a growing tendency to teach entrepreneurship skills. Such skills have allowed for the emergence of the actor-entrepreneur, who succeeds what Broderick Chow describes as the actor-manager. Chow's historical reading suggests that the 'how to act' actor-training processes resonate with the 'how to get an acting job' processes: both the actor-manager and the Stanislavski actor plan a series of actions and execute them, the first as a socio-economic agent of the acting field and the second as an artistic agent within the same field (Chow 2014: 135). Ultimately, Chow points out that the origin of the actor-manager coincided with the development of organizational management under capitalism (ibid.). Similarly, the emergence of the actor-entrepreneur historically coincides with the last decade's economic changes in the UK acting field and beyond.

Actor-training institutions' focus on the development of the self-employed artist since the 2000s, coincides with the 'growing recognition of the value of the creative industries to the UK's growth and prosperity' (Evans 2010: 1) and the promotion of 'small new businesses and entrepreneurial activity by graduates from across all sectors' (ibid.). Already by 2010, entrepreneurship skills such as setting up companies, raising funds, touring work and 'experiencing the professional environment and life-world of small-scale theatre entrepreneurs and businesses' (Evans 2010: 30) are embedded in the curriculum and represent a 'holistic, integrated and immersive entrepreneurial experience, highly engaging and strongly motivating for the student' (ibid.). Investing time in entrepreneurship skills promotes the 'employability credentials' of the actor-training institution and perpetuates the idea of the 'hopeful future,' as projected by neo-liberal ideology. The actor-entrepreneur is not only a creator who takes the initiative, and by doing so changes their future, but they are equipped with 'transferrable skills' that guarantee employability in the broader neo-liberal job market. However, the ratio between practice/theory/entrepreneurship shows less focus on entrepreneurship (Evans 2010: 12–15). After the 2008 economic crisis and its consequences for the acting field, if entrepreneurship skills are seen in the light of the great risk that female trainees take willingly, it appears that more actor-training time should be spent on 'getting acting jobs skills.'

Actor-training institutions have varied graduate employment rates, which in the first instance seem to be related to the diversity of the courses' curricula, structures and policies. This might indicate that the curriculums of courses with higher employability rates, like prestigious conservatoires, should be followed as an example. However, such thinking neglects how the actor-training and acting fields sit within the broader social structure of the acting field. Mark Evans in *Movement Training for the Modern Actor* (2009) writes that the actor-training course that an actor graduates from is a form of capital that has an impact on her future career: prestigious training courses can equip the trainee with greater capital and improve their employability. Because of the higher economic expectations of prestigious institutions, including fees and the high cost of living in London where most of these institutions are, trainees with particular resources can afford to enrol on particular courses. Even though various policy bodies pressurize prestigious institutions to become accessible, still the majority of their trainees derive from privileged economic backgrounds: scholarships cannot defeat either the high fees or the high cost of living in London, both of which keep rising with every year. Prior suggests that the prestige of such institutions guarantees better future employability for its already privileged students: they attract the best students, more high-profile teachers, wealthy benefactors, the 'best' agents and the 'best' jobs (2012: 136). Consequently, their trainees can afford to spend less time in 'getting acting jobs skills.'

However, not all trainees graduate from prestigious drama schools and, even if they do, not everyone achieves agent representation (Prior 2012: 79). The trainee hopes that the training will transfer her from non-professional life to the professional life, but the idea that time in training alone guarantees work is an illusion. Therefore, not only does the trainee actor not invest in her human capital, which will return earnings on graduation, but she is more likely to be the one who sponsors the institution, and in the long-term the acting field. The experience of buying time in actor training as a 'commodity of illusion' with the future hope of an acting career puts the trainee into a place where the chasing of the dream, or the carrot, turns her into an unconscious sponsor of the field.

Conclusion: the commodity of illusion and the neo-liberal hopeful future

There are clear problems with the idea that time in actor-training is preparation for work and that investment in human capital will return money to the female trainee. UK actor-training institutions ought to consider the material realities of the acting profession in the neo-liberal economy and the ethical implications of using the term 'employability'. At the moment, institutions fail to address the inequalities of the acting market, and their employability agenda does not address the fact that women are less desirable actor-training products. Individual trainees cannot see the problem as systemic and institutionalized because it is often reduced to an individual level: 'you are just not good enough'.

If employability is increasingly associated with entrepreneurship, then prioritizing the skills of the actor-entrepreneur would be beneficial for the trainee's socio-economic prospects. I would suggest that embracing the new organizational structure which sees actor-training institutions/trainees as businesses/consumers can prompt female trainees to explore the capitalist system for their own benefit. Fighting the inequalities in the acting field with tools that were developed within the mechanisms of the capitalist system has a potential of working within the system to reform actor-training and the industry. I therefore suggest that time in actor training should be invested both in acting and entrepreneurship skills, with an entrepreneurial environment being a priority in non-prestigious actor-training institutions.

The implementation of the actor-entrepreneur further sustains the neo-liberal agenda of the field by sustaining its existence and prosperity. To continue to produce for the saturated neo-liberal acting market, it is essential to focus in the present and have faith in the future. The fact that women are less desirable than men not only affects the individual's agency and well-being but also causes a specific form of crisis in the market. The identification of specific actors as less desirable leads to two options: either stop the production line of "other actors" – which many training courses do by recruiting only people who look, sound and move in specific desirable ways – or invite actors to create their own future. Until there is a systematic effort to address the inequalities in the acting industry, time in actor-training for women remains a commodity of illusion. Sphinx Theatre uses the Bechdel Test for stage with the aim to 'encourage theatre-makers to think how to write more and better roles for women' (Snow 2015). Similarly, policy bodies ought to develop tools that investigate how the unequal experience of time affects the agency and well-being of female trainees and encourage actor-training institutions to take positive action.

Notes

1 Purple Seven is an audience insight agency that analyses data in the Arts and Entertainment industry. It collects data from 110 venues across the UK, including the Barbican and Sadler's Wells (www.purpleseven.co.uk). Its 'Gender in Theatre' study is 'powered by the largest survey of UK theatregoers with half a million responses and is designed for venues to precisely target marketing and identify the diversity in their audiences' (Purple Seven 2015). The study highlights the paradox that even though women account for 65% of audiences, 'only 39% of actors, 36% of directors and 28% or writers' are women (ibid.).

2 If I were analysing actor training from a cultural rather than a socio-economic perspective, it would be more appropriate to use Pierre Bourdieu's notion of academic capital, rather than Becker's human capital. Academic capital relates to a person's formal education and is measured by their degrees or diplomas and is not reducible to economic capital (Bourdieu 1993: 7). However, there are two problems with using Bourdieu's concept in a discussion of time and temporality. First, it relates only to qualifications, rather than the process of training, which is an experience of time. Second, conservatoires and institutions in the UK over the past decade have been operating as hybrid structures combining educational and corporate objectives and modes of functioning. This makes the trainee actor's academic capital of a different kind to that which Bourdieu discussed, and more relevant to professionalization and turning the investment into money.

3 For example, Becker writes that incomes tend to be higher for urban white males than for black rural males, and higher for black women than for white (2009: 9). The relationship between education and earnings is more complicated when it comes to minorities, with women and minorities earning less than white men when they show 'lower productivity signals' – for example when they hold a degree which they acquired after three years of study – and more than white men when they show higher productivity signals – for example when they are accredited by specific professional bodies (Belman and Heywood 1991: 720). The difference in earnings also vary depending on the specific subjects undertaken. For example, 'women undertaking education, economics, accountancy or law subjects have significantly higher returns to their higher education than women undertaking other subjects' (Blundell et al. 1999: 13).

4 According to 'UCAS conservatoire end of cycle 2016: acceptances by sex' data, the number of applicants accepted into conservatoires rose from 1,355 in 2010 to 2,250 in 2016. Of the 2,250 trainees who were accepted into conservatoires in 2016, 55.3% were women and 44.7% were men. The 55.3% represents 23% of the total number of women applicants, whereas the 44.7% represents the 31% of the total number of men applicants (UCAS 2016a).

5 The equation is very similar for Postgraduate applications and acceptances (UCAS 2016d: 40–42).

6 Purple Seven suggests that this is due to the majority of writers being men (2014).

7 Alison Bechdel's comic strip 'The Rule' sets out two questions to probe the gender inequality in movies: Does the movie contain at least two women? Do they talk to each other about something other than a man? (Bechdel 1985). The Bechdel test aims to raise awareness of, and tackle issues relating to, the representation of women in the media, but it can also be used for theatre works.

8 If this was a cultural analysis rather than a materialist feminist one, Bourdieu's concept of capital could lead us to think that the incentive of most trainee actors, especially women, is non-monetary. Trainees may aim to maximize what Bourdieu describes as their cultural and social capital, which are immaterial (1986: 241–58). Cultural capital comprises the individual's cultural goods and consumption, and their social connections. Applying this to the actor-training environment, trainees would seem to be aiming to advance their cultural goods and consumption, and their social connections.

References

Bechdel, A. (1985) 'Dykes to watch out for,' *Funny Times*, Ohio: Susan Wolpert and Raymond Lesser.

Becker, G. (2009) *Human Capital: A Theoretical and Empirical Analysis with Special Reference to Education*, 3rd ed., Chicago, IL and London: University of Chicago Press.

Belman, D. and Heywood, J.S. (1991) 'Sheepskin effects in the returns to education: an examination of women and minorities,' *The Review of Economics and Statistics*, 73(4): 720–24.

Blundell, R., Dearden, L., Meghir, C. and Sianesi, B. (1999) 'Human capital investment: the returns from education and training to the individual, the firm and the economy,' *Fiscal studies*, 20(1): 1–23.

Bourdieu, P. (1993) *The Field of Cultural Production: Essays on Art and Literature*, Cambridge: Polity Press.

——— (1986) 'The forms of capital,' in Richardson, J. (ed.) *Handbook of Theory and Research for the Sociology of Education*, New York: Greenwood Press, 241–58.

Brecht, B. and Anderson, E. (1961) 'Theatre for learning,' *The Tulane Drama Review*, 6(1): 18–25.

Camilleri, F. (2009) 'Of pounds of flesh and trojan horses: performer training in the twenty-first century,' *Performance Research*, 14(2): 26–34.

Chow, B. (2014) 'An actor manages: actor training and managerial ideology,' *Theatre, Dance and Performance Training*, 5(2): 131–43.

Competition & Markets Authority. (2015a) 'Undergraduate students: your rights under consumer law,' https://www.gov.uk/government/uploads/system/uploads/attachment_data/file/415732/Undergraduate_students_-_your_rights_under_consumer_law.pdf (Accessed 21 Septmeber 2017).

——— (2015b) 'Higher education: consumer law advice for providers', https://www.gov.uk/government/publications/higher-education-consumer-law-advice-for-providers (Accessed 21 September 2017).

Evans, M. (2009) *Movement Training for the Modern Actor*, London: Routledge.

——— (2010) *Making Theatre Work: Entrepreneurship and Professional Practice in Theatre Higher Education*, Lancaster: PALATINE. https://www.heacademy.ac.uk/knowledge-hub/making-theatre-work-entrepreneurship-and-professional-practice-higher-education.

Harvey, A. (2015) 'Funding arts and culture in a time of austerity,' *Arts Council England*, http://www.artscouncil.org.uk/sites/default/files/download-file/Funding%20Arts%20and%20Culture%20in%20a%20time%20of%20Austerity%20(Adrian%20Harvey).pdf (Accessed 28 September 2017).

Harvie, J. (2009) *Theatre & the City, Theatre*, London: Palgrave Macmillan.

Hodge, A. (2000) *Twentieth-Century Actor Training*, London: Routledge.

HM (Her Majesty's) Treasury. (2010) 'Spending review 2010,' October 2010, https://www.gov.uk/government/uploads/system/uploads/attachment_data/file/203826/Spending_review_2010.pdf (Accessed 28 September 2017).

Kapsali, M. (2014a) 'Editorial,' *Theatre, Dance and Performance Training*, 5(2): 103–6. 'Employer and student perspectives on employability'.

——— (2014b) 'Training in a cold climate: edited transcript of roundtable discussion with Catherine Alexander, Alison Andrews, Tom Cornford, Matt Hargrave, Struan Leslie, Kylie Walsh,' *Theatre, Dance and Performance Training*, 5(2): 219–32.

Prior, R.W. (2012) *Teaching Actors: Knowledge Transfer in Actor Training*, Bristol, UK and Chicago, USA: Intellect Books.

Purple Seven. (2014) 'Mind the gender gap,' http://www.purpleseven.com/media.ashx/uktheatremagazinedigitalonline.pdf (Accessed 28 September 2017).

———— (2015) 'Gender in theatre,' http://purpleseven.com/media.ashx/gender-thought-leadership.pdf (Accessed 13 September 2017).

Quality Assurance Agency for Higher Education. (2015) 'Subject benchmark statement: dance drama and performance,' http://www.qaa.ac.uk/en/Publications/Documents/SBS-Dance-Drama-Performance-15.pdf (Accessed 21 September 2017).

Ridout, N. (2014) *Passionate Amateurs: Theatre, Communism and Love*, Ann Arbor: University of Michigan Press.

Simkins, M. (2009) 'When the going gets tough,' *Guide to Performing: Acting*, http://www.theguardian.com/stage/2009/may/09/tips-surviving-acting-industry (Accessed 13 September 2017).

Snow, G. (2015) 'Theatre gets its own Bechdel Test,' News, *The Stage*, 30 November 2015, https://www.thestage.co.uk/news/2015/theatre-gets-its-own-bechdel-test/. (Accessed 13 September 2017).

Tibby, M. (2012) 'Briefing paper for teaching and learning summit on employability,' *The Higher Education Academy*, http://www.agcas.org.uk/assets/download?file=3630&parent=1399 (Accessed 21 September 2017).

UCAS. (2015) 'Conservatoires: end of cycle 2014 report,' https://www.ucas.com/file/21066/download?token=0eP_O3J4 (Accessed 13 September 2017).

———— (2016a) 'Conservatoires end of cycle 2016 data resources: acceptances by sex,' https://www.ucas.com/file/107141/download?token=5WpMW6XL (Accessed 13 September 2017).

———— (2016b) 'Conservatoires: end of cycle 2015 report,' https://www.ucas.com/file/62881/download?token=OnRaBaAy (Accessed 13 September 2017).

———— (2016c) 'End of cycle 2016 data resources: acceptances by detailed subject group and sex,' https://www.ucas.com/file/84376/download?token=VJU5c7dy (Accessed 13 September 2017).

Vincent, A. (2014) 'More than half of actors are under poverty line,' *The Telegraph*, http://www.telegraph.co.uk/culture/theatre/theatre-news/10574735/More-than-half-of-actors-are-under-poverty-line.html (Accessed 14 September 2017).

Willmott, P. (2015) 'Phil Willmott: what should we tell young actresses?' *The Stage*, https://www.thestage.co.uk/opinion/2015/phil-willmott-tell-young- actresses/ (Accessed 14 September 2017).

SECTION III

On time

Temporalizing time through technique

7

THE ECOLOGY OF A SENSE OF GOOD TIMING

Darren Tunstall

We often think we can sense good timing in the telling of a joke or in a moment of drama. At the same time, we also think that every performer has their own special timing. How do we reconcile this apparent contradiction? Where do we get the belief in a sense of timing from? Is good timing only in the mind of the individual – either the performer or the beholder? If so, it's presumably a matter of taste. If not, what evidence could a performer draw upon to improve their timing? This chapter will consider findings from behavioural and movement science, relate them to an established model from social cognitive psychology, suggest relationships to theatre practice and training and propose avenues for future research.

What is timing?

According to the *OED*, there are at least seven distinguishable uses of the English word *timing*. From around 1300, it referred to the fact of an event occurring, but with an additional sense of good fortune or opportunity: it had a moral and emotional component. From the Renaissance onwards, timing became associated with the notion of a performance or a choice. Around 1575 (especially in the humanist disciplines of music and oratory), it came to refer to the action of singing or speaking at, or according to, a specific time (i.e. a rhythmical measure). From 1647, it took on a more general sense of a choice regarding when something should be done so as to maximize one's chances of achieving one's aims. Around 1859, this sense of choice was extended to sport, particularly cricket, where timing came to mean the control of the speed and moment of execution of a stroke through movement coordination. Three points of relevance to this chapter emerge from these definitions:

1. Timing has a moral and emotional component;
2. Timing is a matter of a choice or a performance;
3. Timing relates to coordination of movement for a desired effect.

How can it be measured?

To analyse timing properly, we have to separate the signal – the behaviour – from the surrounding noise. The noise is the range of small, usually unintentional movements of the body that may accompany one's larger actions in the moment, for instance when a task is cognitively demanding. A related problem is that human behaviour is not always made up of single movements in isolation, but often consists of clusters of movements. So, is it better to single out a particular movement from the cluster or to take the cluster as a whole?

One solution to the problem is to consider the goal of the movement. If I scratch my nose with my finger, there may be some accompanying movement that enters into the picture as noise, but the purpose is clear. We could take such a movement as a single unit of action, while any movement that doesn't serve that purpose would be considered separately if at all, and that helps to control the variables somewhat – although there is always a degree of noise or variability in the execution of any movement.

How are the units structured?

The next step is to consider how these action units are structured temporally: is this a purely subjective structuring, or are there universal properties of the brain that produce temporal structure? Many psychologists and psychophysicists, such as Ernst Pöppel, Jacques Michon, Richard Block and Paul Fraisse, have argued that the brain requires a time window to process contextual information. This window has been defined as 'the time interval in which sensory information and concurrent behaviour are to be integrated within the same span of attention' (London 2004: 30); it constitutes a temporal platform for consciousness. Fraisse suggested an average of two to three seconds, with an upper limit of five seconds, as the duration of this time window (Fraisse 1984: 9–10). In other words, every two to three seconds, we segment reality into integrated 'pictures of the present' (ibid: 88). The common name for this temporal integration is the *psychological present*.

The psychological present – the moment of processing the stream of information that constitutes our environment – is not a continuous event in spite of our feeling that it is. Instead, the brain packages the continuous stream of sensory information and internal responses into discrete units so that we can then decide what to do next – such as store this information in longer-term memory, or make a prediction, or a decision, or take an action, or simply discard the information as not worth keeping in one's memory (which is what we actually do with most of it). The brain is essentially turning a stream of sensory data into a chunk of meaning. The three-second window of temporal integration, as it is known, is how everyone perceives the world around them. In fact, we may well share this perceptual binding of events into a subjective present with higher mammals (Pöppel 1997: 59).

How does this structure relate to our perception of timing?

If we create these time windows in our own minds, then it would make sense that we are capable of perceiving manifestations of them in the behaviour of others, even if this occurs below the threshold of our immediate awareness, because it would help us read another person's intentions. I suggest that this capacity forms the basis of our feeling that someone has a good (or bad) sense of timing. It is partly because of our experiential sense of the psychological present, for instance, that we are able to perceive that there is such a thing as rhythm. By rhythm I mean the perception of a sense of order in the stream of data from the environment (or from within our bodies, as with a heartbeat). We perceive the repetition of a stimulus within a given interval. We pick out repeated stimuli and call them *accents*. What we are doing, as the music theorist Justin London argues, is directing attentional energy to a point in time – or rather, to an event that occurs at that point. We project a sense both of temporal location and of salience onto that event (London 2004: 23). Thus, it is that we are able to define a pattern in time and anticipate future stimuli. This capacity to perceive a pattern within a set of stimuli, and thereby to make predictions about the pattern, is at its simplest what rhythm means. A grouping of discrete elements into a perceived rhythm is one example of the durational process by which we apprehend and link together a set of objects to form a kind of narrative of 'what is happening now,' as it were.

What evidence exists for this structure?

Evidence for temporal integration was gathered by Schleidt and Kien (1997). It is their concept of an 'action unit' that I have borrowed for this chapter. They analysed 1,542 action units drawn from five different cultural groups. They found that 93% of the action units they analysed took between two to three seconds. The principle applies to both voluntary gestures and involuntary movements like fidgeting. Some people of course seem to move more quickly or slowly than others as a rule. In this case, they will usually still try to incorporate their movements within a given action unit, thereby confirming the three-second principle (Schleidt 1988). The research finding that most intentional gestures are two to three seconds long includes gestures-for-speaking, since they are timed to synchronize with speech and speaking itself 'is embedded in temporal windows of up to 3 seconds duration giving speech its rhythmic structure' (Pöppel 2004: 300). Thus, not only do we *perceive* using a three-second default principle, we tend to *behave* in accordance with it as well. When we come to talk about emotions, we may find that displays of, say, frustration, anger or excitement result in more and quicker body movements. The person begins to look agitated. How are we able to tell this, unless we have a measuring stick? And the measuring stick, in this case, is a model of rhythmic behaviour determined by the three-second window of the psychological present. This is how we understand a person to be in a state of relative homeostasis: their movements fit into the window. Of course, there are contextual factors to take into account, such as a person's habitual rhythmicity or 'spontaneous tempo,' but this does not contradict the principle – it merely confirms it, because we define a quality like 'quickly' with reference to the three-second window. By way of further illustration, Scott Fairhall and colleagues noted that 'although the duration of individual shots in Hollywood films varies greatly, it is rare to find shots less than around 2 seconds,' probably because

> event information is accumulated over a period of a few seconds, making clip durations of 2–3 seconds an ideal compromise between efficiency (showing as many different shots as possible in a short period of time) and ease of viewing.
>
> *(Fairhall et al. 2014: 5)*

By 'ease of viewing,' the authors are referring to the fluency with which information can be processed mentally; the concept of efficiency will be addressed later in this chapter.

Are there other factors influencing this structure?

Another fundamental principle behind human movement is biomechanical efficiency. I don't mean that every single move we make in any given environmental context is efficient; clearly that isn't the case. I mean that bodily efficiency is adaptive: it has evolved to operate like a default setting. Whenever possible, in order to safeguard its well-being, the human body reverts to homeostasis – it carries out a complex set of internal interactions to maintain or return the body to stable physical and psychological functioning. To achieve homeostasis, you must seek an optimum trade-off between effort and reward – you must use your energy efficiently (see, for instance, Cordain et al. 1997; Critchley 2005; Porges 2009).

How does efficiency manifest in the movement itself – are there formal properties of the movement that can be generalized across different contexts? I think there are, and they relate to a sense of good timing. For example, Tamar Flash and Neville Hogan have outlined a mathematical model of 'maximum smoothness.' They state that 'voluntary movements are made to be as smooth as possible under the given circumstances, at least in the absence of any other overriding concern' such as the need to move fast in the situation (Flash and Hogan: 170). The human motor system tries to achieve maximally smooth movements. Smoothness is measured here in terms of 'jerk,' which refers to the rate of change of acceleration. The smoothest movement is the one that minimizes the quantity of jerk. Assuming a movement that begins at rest in one position and ends at rest in another, then a bell-shaped curve has been shown experimentally many times to pertain for voluntary movements in primates (Nelson 1983; Flash and Hogan 1987; Burdet and Milner 1998; Todorov and Jordan 1998; Flash and Hochner

2005). If you calculate the average velocity of the movement (velocity means speed in a certain direction), and then you work out the peak velocity, i.e. the fastest speed in a certain direction that the movement achieves, you can derive a ratio of peak velocity to average velocity. Hogan found that for 'movements of different amplitudes and durations, the ratio of peak speed to average speed was invariant at 1.88. For a repetitive sequence of movements, speed profiles were again symmetric and this ratio was again invariant, but with a value of 1.57' (Flash et al. 2003: 828). So, at its fastest point, a smooth movement in a given direction is almost – but not quite – twice as fast as its average velocity, and for repeated movements, just over one-and-a-half times as fast. Flash and Hogan (1985) show that the model extends beyond single movements into multi-joint motions and from straight motions to curved ones.

When other concerns become prioritized due to context, such as speed, accuracy or force, it becomes possible to produce a measure of deviation. Even more interesting, though, is that asymmetric velocity profiles are more characteristic of discrete, goal-directed movements as opposed to rhythmically repeated movements. That's because we gravitate towards homeostasis, and a goal-directed movement is usually carried out in an effort to get closer to homeostasis, i.e. in a context where homeostasis is relatively absent.

How do these other factors relate to our perception of timing?

Velocity profiles may suggest one way that we read a person's intentions. Cristina Becchio and colleagues in a number of experiments have shown that individuals can read social intentions from the kinematics of movement alone. A point-light display that provides only minimal information on the joint movements of an arm as it reaches for an object gives sufficient data for subjects to anticipate whether the person will reach for the object with an intention to cooperate, compete or perform an individual action with it. Competitive behaviour was readily associated in their research with a fast speed, and cooperative behaviour with a more natural speed (see Becchio et al. 2012). Your motor system does not simply react to the sight of another person's movement – it uses its own motor experience to predict the intention behind that movement (within the first 500 ms – half a second – of the movement). It could not do this without a feel for what is a natural, i.e. a default, speed for the movement. This lends further support to the idea that there may be a kind of 'neutral point' available to human movements, at least in this limited biomechanical sense.

Are there other constraints upon our perception of timing?

The principle of minimum jerk is most salient at the boundaries, i.e. the start and end points of the movement. To clarify here what I mean by boundaries: Marr and Vaina (1982) showed that a movement sequence can be decomposed into motion segments. These motion segments are bounded by more or less static states, producing a tripartite structure ('state–motion–state'). The movement segment is thus discrete: 'it has an unambiguously identifiable start and stop; *discrete* movements are bounded by *distinct* postures' (Hogan and Sternad 2007: 16). This general principle may resonate with practitioners and teachers familiar with movement systems for performer training.[1] It is also a standard model deployed in sports sciences for breaking a movement (such as a javelin throw) into discrete segments for analysis: preparation–execution–rest.

But perhaps the perception of boundaries is itself purely subjective? Here again, the evidence suggests otherwise. Newtson and Engquist (1976) demonstrated that perceived event boundaries (which they called 'breakpoints') coincide with sudden changes of behaviour. People are remarkably consistent not only in segmenting observed motion events but also in viewing breakpoints as the most intelligible or salient aspect of the movement. Consistency of segmentation happens regardless of the specific interpretation people give to the motion event; that is, we perceive the boundaries of units of action in the same way whether or not we agree about the goal of the action. Nonetheless, Newtson and Engquist argued that the breakpoint serves not only as a demarcation point but as a kind of summary of the *meaning* of the segment. In other words, even if I don't agree with you on what the movement signified, I will agree with you that the breakpoint is where the meaning landed. What matters is how the movement is begun and how it is completed. Rubin and Richards (1985) extended this work on motion segments. They viewed visible motion boundaries as marked by a brief application of force constituting a start and a stop or a discontinuity such as a change of speed and/or direction. The negotiation of physical breakpoints at the boundary of an action is critical to both the feeling and the meaning of smoothness.

What role is played by the wider social context?

Of course, to 'story' one's experiences in this way is not a value-free activity. It is emotionally and morally charged; that is to say, movement is driven by *affect*. Affect is the most basic form of feeling. It is, very simply, the often unconscious sense that something is either good or bad. The sense of good or bad is related to homeostasis, the feeling that your psychological and physiological well-being is paramount (Craig 2009). Clearly, feelings of good or bad are not always and only internal: they are *social*. That's what I refer to by using the word 'ecology' in the title of this chapter: ecology is the study of interactions between organisms (such as people) and their environment (which of course includes other people). Timing is not just something you have; it is something you display, something you negotiate, something you share.

To both support and extend the idea of the moral–affective aspect of timing, I turn now to research that has been accumulated over the last 50 years by many social psychologists, notably including Susan Fiske (Fiske et al. 2007), Andrea Abele (Abele 2003) and Bogdan Wojciszke (Abele and Wojciszke 2007; 2014).

This research looks at the basic dimensions of social cognition, and concerns itself with schemas, stereotypes, attributions and the like. Many social psychologists have come to a general agreement that there are two dimensions of social cognition, which often go under the name of *agency* (or competence) and *communion* (or warmth). Agency relates to the achievement of individual goals, while communion is a matter of social relations – but of course there's some overlap between them. In essence, these dimensions make sense of two fundamental questions that must be answered in any encounter between (minimally) two persons:

1. What are your intentions towards me? Are they beneficial or harmful? In other words, are you an opportunity or a threat?
2. Are you actually capable of carrying out the opportunity or the threat suggested by your behaviour?

How does this relate to a person's behavioural timing? To answer that, we must return to the idea of smoothness. Smoothness is a quality of movement that is often felt to signal an attractive, trustworthy or competent person. It is a key to managing one's social relationships because it constitutes a set of discreet bodily signals that people respond to when conferring judgment upon the individual who displays it. To put it simply, the completion of the three parts of a movement phrase, executed with an appropriately economical amount of force, is taken as a signal of both warmth and competence. It's not hard to see why: if your peak velocity is more than twice your average velocity, such jerkiness can easily be like an alarm signal to my visual perception. I automatically ask: why are you moving that fast? And if your movement is in my direction, that can be even more alarming, depending upon other contextual factors such as my level of physical self-confidence. Smoothness of movement in fact answers to both components of social cognition: it signals both agency and communion – competence and warmth. (For a discussion of smoothness in relation to acting, see Tunstall 2016; for a historicizing critique of the aesthetics of efficiency, see Evans 2009).

Summary

1. The three-second window of temporal integration is a default structure upon which our perception of timing is built.
2. Smoothness of movement, which is partly an outcome of temporal integration, is a preferred mode of behaviour for actor and observer because it associates with homeostasis.
3. Homeostasis is a physical and psychological necessity with direct consequences for social morality through its connection to affect.
4. Social morality has two primary components: warmth/communion and competence/agency.
5. Smoothness of movement answers to both components: warmth and competence.

What about stylization?

I have looked at a range of evidence in support of an objective, or at least psychologically sufficient, concept of 'good timing' derived from the three-second window of the psychological present, and subject to the constraints of the principle of smoothness. It needs to be said that no kind of movement is to be automatically discounted as of no value to a performance. Some comic performers make great play with a certain physical jerkiness – Chaplin, for instance. Of course, we tend to admire them all the more for achieving remarkable physical feats without breaking their bones, and to that extent there is always somewhere in the performance a sense that they have some degree of self-control. This leads us into considering the stylization of actors' movement. Everyone knows that in some movement disciplines there is a conscious regard for a kind of stylized movement that takes the form of abstracted duration. A number of practices may spring to mind such as Meyerhold's Biomechanics, the choreography of Robert Wilson or Butoh. The goal of this abstracted duration is often to extract desirable features of the behaviour from the overall background of movement, and to extend the physical (and, it is argued, expressive) possibilities of these features. For instance, a movement may be slowed down in Meyerhold's Biomechanics in order that its component parts may be better understood. It is also known that slowing down movement enhances the perception of intentionality (Caruso et al. 2016). Nevertheless, comprehension of, say, an étude by Meyerhold begins with perceived natural features of the movement – the necessary combination of muscle efforts for throwing a stone, for instance (see Pitches 2003). However extended the movement may be, the perception of its timing will be against the kind of psychological background that is subject to the principles that I have been outlining: the three-second window and the principle of efficiency leading to smoothness. Whenever an intentional action, with its tripartite structure (state-motion-state), is carried out beneath or beyond this temporal threshold, there is an immediate feeling that what you're looking at is not simply unselfconscious everyday behaviour. This may well constitute part of the difficulty of carrying off such movements. It's not just that the muscle exertions are hard and strange – it's that the timing is hard and strange as well because it attempts to push against the three-second window. And this may become more or less significant. To execute an action unit, such as scratching your nose in half the preferred time may create surprise, whereas to execute it in twice the preferred time may create suspense.

What avenues for future research are there?

There are a number of possible avenues for further research into theatre training and practice that suggest themselves. One might test audience preferences for more or less smooth movements within a scene, for example. Eye tracking movements could be used to test variations in timing. Motion capture data has already been deployed for a number of different purposes such as dance notation; here, one could manipulate imagery to test the relationship between smoothness and dimensions of social cognition. The connecting thread between these suggested lines of inquiry is the gathering of data on human behaviour that would support practical work on the actor's movement. Such research would invite a truly interdisciplinary approach, in which performing arts practitioners and scholars would join forces with behavioural scientists. I think the time is right for such interdisciplinary work.

My hope is that the evidence I have presented and the inferences I have been drawing from it will resonate with practitioners and teachers who find their own points of connection with some of the terms and ideas I've described. To that end, I can recall many of the exercises and games I have learned from others, such as the clown and mask expert John Wright, that were geared towards a group feeling of good timing. John would always refer what improvisers were doing to the group, which acts as the audience. For instance, in one simple but potent exercise, the performer enters into the space and waits for a response. Often, nothing much happens. He or she then tries something; the audience responds by clapping heartily, or a little bit, or not at all. The performer is trying to understand what the audience wants by reacting to their reaction, allowing its intensity to guide the improvisation (for this and similar games, see Wright 2006). When this is successful, as the performer and the audience become more entrained to each other's psychological present, a feeling grows in the room that the performer is discovering not only their timing but their stage presence, whose components are both rhythmic and ethical – because presence is a matter of both agency (competence) and of communion (warmth). On that point, I return to a central theme of this chapter: that timing is not merely personal, but is irreducibly social.

Note

1 Readers may see a connection, for example, with Vsevolod Meyerhold's description of a movement phrase as *otkaz-posil'-tochka* (see Pitches 2003: 55), or with the 15th-century Noh master Zeami Motokiyo's expression *jo-ha-kyu* (see Oida and Marshall 1997: 30–5).

References

Abele, A.E. (2003) 'The dynamics of masculine–agentic and feminine–communal traits: findings from a prospective study,' *Journal of Personality and Social Psychology*, 85(4): 768–76.

Abele, A. and Wojciszke, B. (2007) 'Agency and communion from the perspective of self versus others', *Journal of Personality and Social Psychology*, 93(5): 751–63.

——— (2014) 'Communal and agentic content in social cognition: a dual perspective model,' in Zanna, M.P. and Olson, J.M. (eds) *Advances in Experimental Social Psychology, Volume 50*, Burlington, MA: Academic Press, 195–255.

Becchio, C., Manera, V., Sartori, L., Cavallo, A. and Castiello, U. (2012) 'Grasping intentions: from thought experiments to empirical evidence,' *Frontiers in Human Neuroscience*, 6(117): 1–6.

Burdet, E. and Milner, T.E. (1998) 'Quantization of human motions and learning of accurate movements,' *Biological Cybernetics*, 78: 307–18.

Caruso, E.M., Burns, Z.C. and Converse, B. (2016) 'Slow motion increases perceived intent,' *Proceedings of the National Academy of Sciences*, 113(33): 9250–55.

Cordain, L., Gotshall, R.W. and Eaton, S.B. (1997) 'Evolutionary aspects of exercise,' in Simopoulos, A.P. (ed.) *World Review of Nutrition and Dietetics 81: 'Nutrition and Fitness: Evolutionary Aspects, Children's Health, Programs and Policies,'* Basel: Karger, 49–60.

Craig, A.D. (Bud). (2009) 'Emotional moments across time: a possible neural basis for time perception in the anterior insula,' *Philosophical Transactions of the Royal Society B*, 364: 1933–42.

Critchley, H.D. (2005) 'Neural mechanisms of autonomic, affective, and cognitive integration,' *The Journal of Comparative Neurology*, 493(1): 154–66.

Evans, M. (2009) *Movement Training for the Modern Actor*, New York and Abingdon: Routledge.

Fiske, S.T., Cuddy, A.J.C. and Glick, P. (2007) 'Universal dimensions of social cognition: warmth and competence,' *Trends in Cognitive Sciences*, 119(2): 77–83.

Flash, T. and Hochner, B. (2005) 'Motor primitives in vertebrates and invertebrates,' *Current Opinion in Neurobiology*, 15(6): 660–66.

Flash, T. and Hogan, N. (1985) 'The coordination of arm movements: an experimentally confirmed mathematical model,' *The Journal of Neuroscience*, 5(7): 1688–1703.

—— (1987) 'Moving gracefully: quantitative theories of motor coordination,' *Trends in Neurosciences*, 10(4): 170–74.

Flash, T., Hogan, N. and Richardson, M.J.E. (2003) 'Optimization principles in motor control,' in Arbib, M.A. (ed.) *The Handbook of Brain Theory and Neural Networks, Second Edition*, London and Cambridge, MA: MIT Press.

Fraisse, P. (1984) 'Perception and estimation of time,' *Annual Review of Psychology*, 35: 1–37.

Hogan, N. and Sternad, D. (2007) 'On rhythmic and discrete movements: reflections, definitions and implications for motor control,' *Experimental Brain Research*, 181: 13–30.

London, J. (2004) *Hearing in Time: Psychological Aspects of Musical Meter*, Oxford: OUP.

Marr, D. and Vaina, L. (1982) 'Representation and recognition of the movements of shapes,' *Proceedings of the Royal Society of London, Series B: Biological Sciences*, 214(1197): 501–24.

Nelson, W.L. (1983) 'Physical principles for economies of skilled movements,' *Biological Cybernetics*, 46: 135–47.

Newtson, D. and Engquist, G. (1976) 'The Perceptual Organization of Ongoing Behavior', *Journal of Experimental Social Psychology*, 12(5): 436–50.

Oida, Y. and Marshall, L. (1997) *The Invisible Actor*, Abingdon and New York: Routledge.

Pitches, J. (2003) *Vsevolod Meyerhold*, London and New York: Routledge.

Pöppel, E. (1997) 'A hierarchical model of temporal perception,' *Trends in Cognitive Sciences*, 1: 56–61.

—— (2004) 'Lost in time: a historical frame, elementary processing units and the 3-second window,' *Acta Neurobiologiae Experimentalis*, 64: 295–301.

Porges, S.W. (2009) 'The polyvagal theory: new insights into adaptive reactions of the autonomic nervous system,' *Cleveland Clinic Journal of Medicine*, 76 (Suppl. 2): S86–S90.

Rubin, J.M. and Richards, W.A. (1985) 'Boundaries of visual motion,' *Massachusetts Institute of Technology Artificial Intelligence Laboratory, AI Memo 835*, http://publications.ai.mit.edu/ai-publications/pdf/AIM-835.pdf.

Schleidt, M. (1988) 'Universal time constant operating in human short-term behaviour repetitions,' *Ethology*, 77(1): 67–75.

Schleidt, M. and Kien, J. (1997) 'Segmentation in behaviour and what it can tell us about brain function,' *Human Nature*, 8(1): 77–111.

Todorov, E. and Jordan, M.I. (1998) 'Smoothness maximization along a predefined path accurately predicts the speed profiles of complex arm movements,' *Journal of Neurophysiology*, 80(2): 696–714.

Tunstall, D. (2016) *Shakespeare and Gesture in Practice*, Basingstoke and New York: Palgrave Macmillan.

Wright, J. (2006) *Why is that So Funny? A Practical Exploration of Physical Comedy*, London: Nick Hern Books.

8

GATHERING GHOSTS

Lecoq's twenty movements as a technique to mark time

Jenny Swingler

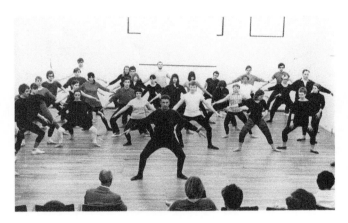

FIGURE 8.1 Jacques Lecoq teaching the twenty movements, 1972. © Collection Ecole Jacques Lecoq.

The twenty movements are a crucial rite of passage in the Lecoq training (see Figure 8.1). Towards the end of the first year, a sacred test is pinned to the wall in the foyer; the colour of deerskin and burnt earth, it is reminiscent of a cave painting or ancient mural and each figurine represents a movement established by Jacques Lecoq himself. Never before were we so clearly faced with the out-stretched hand of the past.

The school is full of ghosts. When entering the building, the students are met with a wall of photographs of past students, dating back to the 1950s. Faces peer and squint out from a brightly-lit photo booth somewhere in the past. The whole thing looks like an appeal for the missing.

Even the building itself is a reminder of that which has come before. Having been a renowned boxing club in the 1930s, the *Grande Salle* reverberates like an architectural testimony to the laws of movement, the push and pull of the fight, the *légèrté* of the win and the tragedy of the knock out.

The twenty movements are a text that was written in the past for an action in the present.

Like a spine in the School's training, the movements are practised throughout the first year and are key to demonstrating the integral dynamics of the body. Weight is required in the motivation of the discus-thrower, the *passeur* embodies the continual circulation of push and pull and the *eclosion*, an integral moment of suspension between maximum expansion and the closing in of the body within the space. The movements are like physical sketches – each engineered as a reminder of the physical body in action. Throughout the training, we are reminded that to deny the dynamics of the moving body is to deny life itself and would lead to a type of theatre that is lacking in life: a dead theatre.

The only time each student is obliged to perform alone before the rest of the School is during the demonstration of the twenty movements at the end of the first year. Here, a discourse arises between each student's present interpretation of the movements and the history of the School. Like a Hamlet soliloquy, there is a sense that the physical text can never be performed without the reverberation of those who have gone before. To commit to a movement forged in the past allows a simultaneous embodiment of a certain liveness which is reborn in the present body of each performer and at the same time, the enduring relevance of the dynamics that can be traced in the body in motion.

Each individual performer cannot help but meet the movements differently and thus the rigid template hanging on the wall is momentarily in flux as multiple interpretations spiral out as students leave momentarily fresh tracks; tracks which will have faded as next year's students begin to trace the movements with their own bodies.

At this point in the training, one develops a sense that the distinct specificity of each performing body is at the forefront of creation. Rather than bonding students to the past, Lecoq insisted that his School was intended to train artists to 'acquire an understanding of acting and develop their imaginations. This allows them either to invent their own theatre or to interpret written texts, if they so desire, but in new ways' (Lecoq 2001: 16).

Indeed, there is a sense on graduating that the invention of a new kind of theatre is possible. In 2011, I co-founded Clout Theatre; as an international ensemble, we were bound by an endeavour to use our training to create our own theatrical language. And yet, a subtle haunting began to permeate our work. We were like teenagers leaving home to carve our own legacy only to find ancestral gestures reverberating through our muscles. Whilst each training has its ghosts, the South American influence upon Grotowski's Theatre of Sources (Schechner 1997) or the trauma of rapid industrialization in post-war Japan that can be traced in Butoh (Nanako 2000: 10–28), it is perhaps only when leaving the training that the form of these ghosts can really begin to emerge.

Mark Evans' research into the possible influences that make up the Lecoq training led him to cite exercises with 'roots in European physical training' and the 'late nineteenth-/early twentieth-century construction of the efficient body' (Evans 2014: 148). I would also add that the presence of the 'efficient body' in Lecoq's twenty movements could perhaps be seen to capture the cultural imprint upon a generation shaped by the impact of war, industrialization and manual labour. Indeed, the French Resistance framed Lecoq's own training, as he attended the Association Travail et Culture (TEC) which created 'cultural opportunities for working class people' during the Resistance (Kemp 2017: 1–8).

The insistence, throughout the training, for the performer to have their heels firmly planted on the ground in the execution of each movement is a detail which I believe captures the way in which the importance of the efficient body remains at the forefront of the training. A seemingly trivial detail, the stability of the body not only ensures neutrality but also indicates a performing body of action and reaction that is permanently bound to an era where the efficient body was exemplified through action. To leave the heel up was a sign of not assuming the movement fully, a suggestion of an inefficiency and inaction as the body is no longer grounded.

As a company exploring the body in performance in the 21st century, our training has at times caused frustration. Through the impact of the training, our instincts as performers are born from a corporeality that is profoundly located in the era in which Lecoq forged his training. It is perhaps no surprise that Lecoq-trained companies can often be found to set initial work after graduating in the fractured landscape of Europe at war. The training has permeated our movements to conjure a post-war world. This can frequently be traced in the various exercises and improvisations throughout the training. When studying melodrama, students are asked to improvise around themes such as 'The Soldier's Return' or 'The Departure for America.'

Thus, through our endeavours to explore inertia in *The Various Lives of Infinite Nullity* (2012) or the mediatized body in *Feast* (2015), our relationship to the twenty movements and the efficient body had become in, and of itself, a continual state of push and pull. The movements remind us both of our common lineage and our shared effort to push against aspects of the training that now feel to be stuck in a post-war era. It could be said that whilst we are happily bound to a training in which the performing body can only be of use if the performer is aware of the principles of movement that are as sustaining as the human body itself, we have decided for now, to occasionally keep our heels up.

References

Evans, M. (2014) 'Playing with history: personal accounts of the political and cultural self in actor training through movement,' *Theatre, Dance and Performance Training*, 5(2): 144–56.

Kemp, R. (2017) 'Jacques Lecoq,' *Digital Theatre: Encyclopedia of Performance*, 1–8. https://www.digitaltheatreplus.com/education/study-guides/jacques-lecoq.

Lecoq, J. (2001) *The Moving Body*, trans. D. Bradby, London: Routledge.

Nanako, K. (2000) 'Introduction: Hijikata Tatsumi: The words of Butoh,' *TDR/The Drama Review*, 44(1): 10–28.

Schechner, R. (1997) *The Grotowski Sourcebook*, New York: Routledge.

9

ADAVU

Drilling through time

Mark Hamilton

I have been dancing *bharatanatyam* (South Indian classical dance) for 30 years. I began training with Chitraleka Bolar in Birmingham. My key apprenticeship was with Priya Sreekumar in Edinburgh (UK), and also in India with her *guru* (master) Nattuvanam Paramsiva Menon (1919–2014) – whose own *guru* was the eminent Meenakshi Sundaram Pillai (1869–1954). I am a 48-year-old, white queer Yorkshireman raised as a Methodist and also a New Zealand citizen, having lived there for 13 years. I offer this lineage and biography to position me and my dancing as explicitly as I can.

The heightened experiences generated through training in *bharatanatyam* have given me an embodied induction to Hindu cosmology. In my apprenticeship, like that of most dancers of the form, the rigorous geometry and rhythms of daily drills called *adavu* were used to perfect my performance. They also engaged me in conceptions of a continuum beyond day-to-day understandings of time. The practical discipline and pedagogical discourse of *bharatanatyam* training introduced me to the potential of an atemporal, spiritual dimension of existence. Writing this chapter, I become aware that this shift has also educated me in concepts that have been used to underwrite Hindu nationalist projects in modern India. My *bharatanatyam* training indicates the global reach of practices promoting Hinduism as much as my escapist desire for an East that is the West's Other. I see my acquisition of an 'exotic' conception of time as a process of acculturation rather than appropriation – that is, my assimilation into a belief structure quite distinct from that into which I was born. My experiences indicate how desires for immersion in a timeless Oriental India align with the discourses of contemporary Hindu supremacist ideologies. I examine this proposition by reviewing my *bharatanatyam* training and through reference to an autobiographical solo work created by Shane Shambhu, a fellow male *bharatanatyam* dancer and my research collaborator of three years. Shane and I both undertook *bharatanatyam* training in the UK and our careers offer perspectives on how encounters with the form have fostered our engagement with an ontology quite different from the dominant conceptions of the Western society in which we live.

Last month, I performed *bharatanatyam* at a London intercultural centre for the sacred arts.[1] I danced an invocation of Ganesha (the god of beginnings) and a *pushpanjali* (offering of flowers) in honour of Devi (the omniscient mother goddess). As my feet slapped on the floor and my body flowed through abstract and representative configurations, a familiar shift occurred in my experience of time. Moving dynamically in the immediate space, pushing incrementally forward into the nascent future, corridors of perception also opened up linking my footfalls and gestures with those I have danced before in diverse past moments and those danced by my teachers, and their teachers, and their teachers' teachers, ad infinitum. On the one hand, distinctions that ordinarily hold apart 'then' and 'now' lessened. This chapter considers how *bharatanatyam* fosters such perceptions through its intertwining of performance with Hindu cosmology, interconnecting immediate embodiment and transcendental concepts – a connection that Hindu Indian nationalism promotes. On the other hand, I consider too how my dancing of *bharatanatyam* ever affirms my particular position in a sociocultural, spatiotemporal continuum.

Throughout my *bharatanatyam* career, I have returned to the *adavu*. Looking back over my life, I see myself in spaces across the world engaging with these elementary drills – on the stage of a Māori community centre in Auckland, in a disused cinema on New Zealand's South Island, in the studios of my current London university located within a royal park. These *adavu* have persisted across time and continued in my life while much else has passed away – jobs, homes, love affairs. Yet, simultaneously, the tangible impossibility of realizing the perfect aesthetic form they promise in my unstable human frame conjures tangible sensations of time's transcendence over all practice; the years roll on and a moment when I completely realize the potential of these *adavu* never arrives.

The instrumental power of *adavu* lies in the use of conscious repetition to gradually reorder a performer's movement preferences and material substance. The dancer's body becomes invested with codified stances, gaits and gestures that have been passed on from generation to generation of Indian artists and increasingly (as my career demonstrates) across borders of ethnicity, nationality and geography. My sustained engagement with *adavu* over three decades has fundamentally changed me. In an article elsewhere, I explain that through my recurrent drilling 'seemingly artificial behaviours now emerge from me as reflexive responses, somewhat unbidden and unconscious, almost as if natural' (Hamilton 2017: 1). Through *adavu*, I have become able to articulate precise sequences of postures called *karana*. I learned to configure my feet, weight, spine and limbs (including finger tips and eyes) to the changing tempo of a pulse beaten out on a wooden block by Priya, my principal teacher. I was taught to render each *adavu* in four speeds, from hyper-slow (requiring strength and control) to maximum speed (requiring release and lightness). Priya also required me to master a spectrum of metres ranging from two to nine beat cycles. This training process, measured for accuracy in centimetres and seconds, reorganized my movements to meet ideal forms. Yet in this exactitude, Priya also asked me to find an ease of flow like that used in the familiar tasks of daily life. The perspicacity and sophistication needed to realize the ideal form and flow of each *adavu* grows steadily, year by year, through sustained practice. At the same time, however, the vigour and stamina needed to continue such athletic labours incrementally decline at the same rate. The geometrical and rhythmical perfection *adavu* seek to realize is a challenge that seems ever just beyond my capacity; my moment of their mastery is an ever-receding point.

I have experienced altered perceptions of time, similar to those evoked through *bharatanatyam* training, during deep engagement with other highly rehearsed physical disciplines. They arise from the conjunction of focused awareness and reflexive action. However, the discourse and conventions enfolding *bharatanatyam* shape such experiences as an embodied engagement with Hindu ontology. Through *bharatanatyam* training, I entered what dancer-scholar Uttara Asha Coorlawala calls the 'religio-aesthetic environment of Indian dance' (Coorlawala 1996: 19). She argues that the Hindu culture in which *bharatanatyam* emerged is intrinsic to the form and that 'decontextualised readings' ignoring this factor distort our understanding of it (Coorlawala 1996: 19). Though I speak directly to *bharatanatyam*'s religio-aesthetics, my dancing and critical analysis of the form are always queer. I am the antithesis of the dominant idealization of a *bharatanatyam* dancer as a Hindu Indian woman. My dancing bends norms of gender and culture and my homosexuality further emphasizes this situation. Queer theorist Kenn Gardner Honeychurch argues that sexual orientation is always implicated in 'higher cognitive functions' (Honeychurch, cite in Dilley 1999: 460). This proposition refutes notions of detached objectivity and promotes what Patrick Dilley calls a reduction 'of the space between position and product, investigator and investigation' (Dilley 1999: 460). My queer criticality acknowledges that desire informs all embodiment and thought. Investigating the perception of time that *bharatanatyam* has taught me must thus be grounded in my particular embodied presence in the form; I question how Hindu cosmology resonates with a queer engagement with the power of performativity.

In Shane's solo, called *Confessions of a Cockney Temple Dancer* (hereafter, *Confessions*),[2] he revisits a key performative instant. Shane repeatedly promises to re-enact his solo professional debut at age 18. He details how he trained for the event and demonstrates *adavu* to narrate his days of *gurukula* (live-in schooling). In the closing section of *Confessions*, Shane dances on stage in front of stuttering technicoloured footage of his debut, projected on a small backdrop. An odd generation gap is conjured; 'Shane today' – interdisciplinary theatre artist – executes his own innovative choreography to the 20-year-old recording of Karnatic (traditional South Indian) music from his debut. We see that his new dance combines a range of movement vocabularies while remaining connected to the *adavu* that shaped him as a *bharatanatyam* dancer. Simultaneously, we see 'Shane then' on

screen, fixed in his careful and dutiful rendering of his teachers' classical choreography that is closely connected in every detail to *adavu*.

Confessions presents 'Shane then' as an East End boy immersed in a Hindu
artistic apprenticeship, in which holistic transformation was the paramount process. As I have written elsewhere (Hamilton 2017: 2), *bharatanatyam* training can
be a form of *tapas* – that is, a spiritual discipline fervently pursued to transcend
domestic and commercial material preoccupations. Here, I refine this analysis by
citing dancer-scholar Nandini Sikand to say that *bharatanatyam* can be *sadhana*; 'a
combination of discipline and practice ideally done with the guidance of a guru.
It is a practice characterized by intention, and is based on the idea that through
repetition and awareness there is a movement towards perfection' (Sikand 2012:
238). The perfection the *bharatanatyam* apprentice seeks is embodiment of ideal
form through the reconciliation of exacting abstraction and human life. Pursuit
of this illusive moment through daily drilling in *adavu* gives rise to strong sensations whose recurrence and potency eclipses much else and subsumes those
domestic routines and occasional unique events by which one might ordinarily
mark time's passage. Consistent practice of *adavu* makes a transfixing thread passing through the variables of days and seasons and years.

Rajiv Malhotra's writing promotes an Indian Hindu ontology. He seeks to
redress contemporary colonialist values he identifies inside and outside India that
define the nation as the West's inferior opposite. In *Being Different: An Indian
Challenge to Western Universalism*, he states that Hindu Indian culture conceives
of classical dance forms such as *bharatanatyam* as spiritual practice 'using movement, sound and emotion to internalize [Hindu] cosmology and epistemology
within the dancer's body' (Malhotra 2013: 77). A *bharatanatyam* apprentice is
ordinarily taught a hereditary repertoire of expressive dances narrating stories of
Hindu deities, representing their forms and actions through postures, gestures
and facial expressions. The apprentice's first repertoire also includes some dances
composed almost wholly of abstract movements, such as *allarippu* in which each
body part it articulated one-by-one. Such dances do not characterize deities but
they do communicate Hindu conceptions. When learning such choreographies,
it is most clear that through *bharatanatyam,* an inherited idealized division and re-
structuring of one's corporeality is taught. To drill in *adavu* and to dance abstract
sequences like *allarippu* is to gradually map connections between one's very body
parts and grand cosmological propositions about time and space.

Ananda Coomaraswamy's *The Dance of Siva* (1918) helped seed a pan-Indian
reverence for the South Indian deity of Nataraja (Siva as Lord of the Dance).
As the tutelary deity of *bharatanatyam*, Nataraja has become today the dancer's
exemplar. Processes of training and performance are viewed as replicating his
cyclical acts of creation, preservation and destruction (Coomaraswamy 1957: 70).
Through this association, perceptions of the intertwining of prehistory, the present instant and an atemporal continuum become interwoven with a dancer's
experience of the ever-becoming of the performative moment. Indeed, *bharatanatyam* can invite dancers to move even beyond understanding performance as an

embodiment of a cyclical Hindu cosmogony and enter the form as a vehicle for experiencing the cessation of all progressions.

When drilling in *adavu* or dancing *bharatanatyam* items, Priya asked me to centre my mind wholly in the rigours and complexities of the dance, these being enough to busy every faculty and capacity. She offered dance training as an active meditation through which absorption in complex rhythmic movement might offer, paradoxically, experience of a transcendental timeless stillness. Such a shift is more widely pursued by Hindu devotees through the practice of *japa*, the meditative repetition of a word, particularly the totalizing sound of ॐ (*Aum*), which is considered the preeminent Sanskrit *aksara* (syllable). Malhotra explains that repeated chanting of this sound is 'designed to dissolve nama-rupa (name and form, and the *context* of name and form) from the mind' (Malhotra 2013: 264; original emphasis). *Japa* evokes detachment from the frameworks by which we perceive manifest time – be it the measures of minutes or millennia. Malhotra describes ॐ (*Aum*) as both symbolically representing and effectively evoking an experience of *pralaya* (dissolution), which Devdutt Pattanaik describes as a state in which the 'past, present and future telescope into each other [and the] serpent of time coils rather than slithers' (Pattanaik 2008: 41). In *History of Indian Cosmogonical Ideas*, Narendra Bhattacharyya says *pralaya* denotes the cosmic instances of cessation and reignition through which one aeon ends and another begins (Bhattacharyya 1971: 90). At the same time, he notes, *pralaya* also signifies the potential in each of us to seat our consciousness outside the progress of our individual biography and beyond all human conceptions of time (Bhattacharyya 1971: 77).

Malhotra encapsulates his analysis of a Hindu conception of time when he proposes that where and how a method of *sadhana* evolves matters much less than its efficacy; he says, 'the *techniques* for achieving embodied enlightenment are what is important – not the history' (Malhotra 2013: 87; original emphasis). Malhotra's Hindu transcendentalism holds that 'historical awareness is nice to have, but is not a "must-have" for achieving an embodied state of divine consciousness' (Malhotra 2013: 62). In *Being Different*, he suggests that Indian Hindu ahistoricism is superior to Western historicism. The latter is founded upon conflicting absolutist Abrahamic narratives, simplistic linear models of scientific causation and covet and persistent racist ideologies of European imperialism. The former rests on a sophisticated cosmogony which acknowledges that 'prior to this universe there was another one, and before that, another, and this series of universes is infinite' (Malhotra 2013: 254). Malhotra's Hindu thought focuses not on tracking chronological time but on escaping the endless layers of cyclical creation and the web of *karma* through which previous states of existence have lasting consequences that interconnect all events. He quotes Richard Lannoy to support his portrayal of Hinduism's determined reach beyond earthly time:

> Contrary to the Islamic and Judeo-Christian traditions, history has no metaphysical significance for either Hinduism or Buddhism. The highest

human ideal is jivan-mukta – one who is liberated from Time. Man, according to the Indian view, must, at all costs, find in this world a road that issues upon a trans-historical and a-temporal plane.

(Lannoy in Malhotra 2013: 57)

My writing here might be seen to privilege modes of epistemology that Malhotra considers intrinsically Western. Opening this chapter, I use my biography, described in cultural and gender political terms, to help expose my relationship to my subject of study. Such positionality can be explained with reference to Daniel Johnston's monograph *Theatre and Phenomenology: Manual Philosophy* (2017). He examines how the influence of Martin Heidegger has led Western scholars, such as me, to accept that: 'All human experience is from a definite standpoint in time, looking to the future, and in a distinctive historical period that will enable its own understanding of Being' (Johnston 2017: 45). Malhotra's analysis implies that Hindu Indian ontology is disconnected from this kind of temporal awareness. Yet, I argue a regard for history is not absent but is complicated in the culture that surrounds *bharatanatyam*.

All hereditary Indian arts centre upon the *guru shishya paramapara* (the chain of oral transmission from teacher to student). In *Confessions*, Shane conveys the sense of custodial responsibility this confers upon *bharatanatyam* dancer. In one section, large images of *hasta mudra* (symbolic hand gestures) are projected on the backdrop while Shane simultaneously demonstrates them. He amplifies their complex forms by performing a distinct *karana* he has created for each one. Then, reciting the names and forming the shapes of *mudras*, he places his hand in those of audience members, as if making personal gifts. *Mudra* are rote learnt by *bharatanatyam* students who copy their teachers until each form can be shaped instantaneously when its name is called out. In *Confessions*, Shane describes his hands, and the *mudra* he forms with them, as being part of a chain of hands forming *mudra* that stretches back into antiquity; these shapes have been passed down – hand-to-hand – from one generation to the next, across the aeon (Figure 9.1).

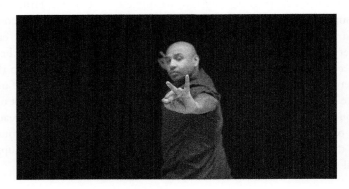

FIGURE 9.1 Shane Shambhu in *Confessions of a Cockney Temple Dancer*. Photo: Simon Richardson.

Mudra, like *adavu*, are treasured by *bharatanatyam* dancers as inheritance from long ago, transmitted by a revered lineage. It is a lineage, however, that is not fully historically elucidated. *Bharatanatyam* is often imagined and mythologized by dancers and audiences of the form (inside and outside of India) as transcendent of any particular chain of direct transmission. There is recourse to a dehistoricizing romanticism that effaces the individual artists whose craft contemporary dancers inherit. Many scholars suggest that this occurs because the history of *bharatanatyam* has been deliberately erased (Apffel-Marglin 1985; Allen 1997; Kersenboom 2011; Soneji 2012). In summary, they argue that the form has been embedded in a version of India's past, manufactured to substantiate the values preferred by the country's modern-day Hindu leadership. Nilanjana Mukherjee recently added to this analysis while contextualizing Rabindranath Tagore's (1861–1941) choreographic innovations (Mukherjee 2017). Mukherjee suggests that, during the early 12th century, upper caste people's revival of Indian arts involved collaboration with nationalist forces to separate hereditary dance practices from matrilineal low-caste communities of temple and court performers. Doing so interrupted longstanding social structures and enacted a strategic appropriation of localized customary practices to serve an emergent elite's national political aims. Mukherjee focuses on how a narrative of classicism decontextualized specific hereditary dance arts and resituated them in what she calls 'a continuum unhindered by sociopolitical or historical changes' (Mukherjee 2017: 86). She proposes that Indian classical dance thus came to represent 'a sanitised Hindu version of India's past and became the repository of "spirituality" which was thought to be lost with years of repeated onslaughts of "foreign" rule' (Mukherjee 2017: 86).

Mukherjee argues that the current spirituality of *bharatanatyam* came into being through a replacement of the form's sociopolitical history with a constructed atemporal frame: the dance has been made a vehicle for the reviving dissemination of a spirituality centred on aspirations considered suitable to support a modern unified and Hindu-centric Indian state. *Bharatanatyam* is thus now posited as *tapas* and *sadhana* promising access to a dimension beyond the material realm through purifying mastery of one's physicality and taking charge of one's embodiment: one's specific spatio-temporal position becomes a means to unlock another world – a gate to a supersensual transcendent dimension. David Smith has examined the historical practices which India's current classicism purports to emulate. In *Hinduism and Modernity*, he notes that despite recent cultural movement away from those very markers, towards new conceptions of a globally informed Indianness, it is always open to the Hindu 'to abandon the social self and become a spiritual self' (Smith 2002: 5).

Bharatanatyam training invites the dancer to surrender to concepts of time-without-end pervading the Hindu cultural continuum the dance ordinarily occupies. The concept of the dance as *sadhana* is upheld by the daily cyclical drills through which it is mastered, the constancy of the mythological narratives which it communicates and the prevalence of dehistoricized descriptions of the form.

In his article 'Politics beyond the Yoga Mat,' Patrick McCartney considers how yoga plays 'an important part in the soft power initiatives of the Indian state' (McCartney 2017: 3). He notes in particular that the 'epistemes and texts, language, and cultural practices' that yoga practitioners 'glorify' are those equally lauded by Hindu supremacists (McCartney 2017: 10). He sees both communities sharing a 'nostalgia for a future-past (similar, perhaps, to a future perfect tense, i.e. "will have")' (McCartney 2017: 2). Participation in yoga, McCartney argues, may make practitioners 'unwitting supporters of an imperialist, Hindu supremacist agenda' (McCartney 2017: 2). McCartney's work raises the possibility that to understand *adavu* as offering an experience of transcending time may also similarly align with supremacist factions favouring a Hindu Indian state. To see *bharatanatyam* as transcendent of time contributes to ideas of Indian culture as overcoming all histories of repression through embodied Hindu practices which access a spiritual power able to erase traces of invasive sociopolitical actions – including Muslim Mogul and Christian British rule.

The releases from time I have experienced through the *sadhana* of *bharatanatyam* are the fruits of a modern cultural practice created alongside the propagation of a modern pan-Indian identity centred on concepts of atemporality as the quintessence of Hinduism's power. Yet in this analysis I do not seek to dismiss the ontology the form has communicated to me. Ashis Nandy, in his essay on the psychology of colonialism, suggests that 'the affirmation of ahistoricity is an affirmation of the dignity and autonomy of non-modern peoples' (Nandy 2009: 59). My life as a *bharatanatyam* dancer attests to the empowering value of an ontology that does not align with Western conceptions. Moreover, Jeremy Carrette's exploration of Foucault's theorizing helps me see that whilst the discourse of any spirituality can never be divorced from the historical continuums it intersects, such discourse can open us to a 'politics of continual transformation by holding up what we can be and what is not yet seen' (Carrette 2013: 71). In *bharatanatyam*, the ideal realization of perfect form ever recedes from attainment and the attainment of spiritual fulfilment always dwells just beyond this material realm. The performative power of the imminent future is twice evoked by the form. Valuing both artistic lineage and atemporal experience, *bharatanatyam* training practices nurture steady growth and can promote radical change in each dancer. I have found personal means of, and innovative self-expression through, my queer deployment of the performative power that this discipline ordinarily utilizes to uphold ideas of tradition.

Adavu practice has altered my body. Over a long time, bodily configurations that once felt strange and artificial have come to flow smoothly. Similarly, through innumerable repetitions of *adavu* and mastery of complex rhythmic patterns, I have become familiar with once-alien and seemingly obscure concepts about an experiential continuum beyond the quotidian. The cyclical cosmogony of Hinduism has infused my world; I have undergone an acculturation. Importantly, this transition has been wrought via immersion in my materiality; drilling in *adavu* involves profuse sweating, blistering heels and specific muscular development. *Bharatanatyam* has become inscribed in my body. But I am a queer dancer of the form standing outside of contemporary Hindu Indian society. I am acculturated but not assimilated. Moreover, my marginal position is made sharper by my increasing awareness of the suppression of hereditary dancer castes and their traditions that has created the modern day form of *bharatanatyam*. My unusual rendering of their dance and my reflective criticism upon this act make explicit the performative processes that evolve the form from moment to moment. My queer embodiment articulates and never escapes the sociopolitical context of my specific spatio-temporal position. Drilling through time has offered me experiences of an ahistorical supra-sensual continuum, but it has simultaneously made me question if any amount of repetitious training can detach anybody from the hold of culturo-historical coordinates.

Notes

1 Daniel P. Cunningham & Mark James Hamilton, *Creatrix: Cosmic Mother* (Colet House, London: 8 July 2017).
2 Shane Shambhu, *Confessions of a Cockney Temple Dancer* (Rich Mix, London: 29 July 2017).

References

Allen, M.H. (1997) 'Rewriting the script for south Indian dance,' *TDR,* 41(3): 63–100.
Apffel-Marglin, F. (1985) *Wives of the God-King: The Rituals of the Devadasis of Puri,* Oxford: Oxford University Press.
Bhattacharyya, N.N. (1971) *History of Indian Cosmogonical Ideas,* New Delhi: Munshiram Manoharlal.
Carrette, J. (2013) 'Rupture and transformation: Foucault's concept of spirituality reconsidered,' *Foucault Studies,* 15: 52–71.
Coomaraswamy, A.K. (1957) *The Dance of Shiva,* New York: Noonday Press.
Coorlawala, U.A. (1996) 'Darshan and abhinaya: an alternative to the male gaze,' *Dance Research Journal,* 28(1): 19–27.
Dilley, P. (1999) 'Queer theory: under construction,' *International Journal of Qualitative Studies in Education,* 12(5), 457–72.
Hamilton, M.J. (2017) 'Ruptures in reformation: embodiment revealed,' *Indian Theatre Journal,* in peer review, 1, 1–16.
Johnston, D. (2017) *Theatre and Phenomenology: Manual Philosophy,* London: Palgrave Macmillan.
Kersenboom, S.C. (2011) *Nityasumangali: Devadasi Tradition in South Asia,* New Delhi: Motilal Banarsidass.
Malhotra, R. (2013) *Being Different: An Indian Challenge to Western Universalism,* Noida: Harper Collins.
McCartney, P. (2017) 'Politics beyond the Yoga Mat: Yoga Fundamentalism and the "Vedic Way of Life",' http://oicd.net/ge/index.php/politics-beyond-yoga-mat-yoga-fundamentalism-vedic-way-life/.
Mukherjee, N. (2017) 'From nautch to nritya,' *Economic and Political Weekly,* 52(3): 85–92.

Nandy, A. (2009) *The Intimate Enemy Loss and Recovery of Self under Colonialism*, Oxford: Oxford University Press.

Pattanaik, D. (2008) *Myth = Mithya*, New Delhi: Penguin.

Sikand, N. (2012) 'Beyond tradition: the practice of sadhana in Odissi dance,' *Journal of Dance & Somatic Practices*, 4(2): 233–47.

Smith, D. (2002) *Hinduism and Modernity*, New Jersey, NJ: Wiley-Blackwell.

Soneji, D. (2012) *Unfinished Gestures: Devadasis, Memory, and Modernity in South India (South Asia Across the Disciplines)*, Chicago, IL: University of Chicago Press.

10

RSVP AND THE TIMELY EXPERIENCE

Gyllian Raby

Devising theatre fits Horst Rittel's definition of a 'wicked' problem, a problem that cuts across categories of knowing, organization, hierarchy and belief (Conklin 2005: 2). Like Rittel, Anna and Lawrence Halprin recognized the need for a process in which the formation of the group and the creation of the work are mutually constitutive, and they created *The RSVP Cycles: Creative Processes in the Human Environment* (1969). Their approach has since been adapted very effectively for the theatre. Practitioners including Jacques Lessard, Robert Lepage and the Commotion youth theatre team, have gravitated to the RSVP cycles. I believe this is partly because extraordinary collective creation flourishes when the joy-killing time pressure exerted by the production schedule – 'the arrow towards perfectibility' – can be sidestepped. Rittel based his solutions for wicked problems on 'morphological analysis' questions that re-shape, disrupt and disjoint the forward pressure of production. In much the same way, the RSVP cycles alter the mental environment of devisers.

There is a debate over whether devising processes draw on the same skills as conventional theatre-making, or whether collective creation is a different animal. Alison Oddey examines 'devised theatre as a separate form' (1994: 1), while James Mackinnon sees devising as contiguous with theatre-making (2015). I suggest that there is a spectrum of devising approaches that range from the 'wicked' to the 'tame.' The extent to which devising benefits from a distinct pedagogy, that is an addition to foundational theatre training, can perhaps be gauged by the extent that a given group addresses their collaboration as a *wicked problem*. The more wicked the problem, the greater the need for a process that engages with diverse creative modes – such as RSVP. The cycles function to disrupt and interrupt the complexity of the wicked problem by immersing participants, knowingly, in different temporal mental environments.

I have worked extensively with various approaches to devising theatre with Canadian companies including One Yellow Rabbit Theatre, Théâtre Repère and my five years on the Commotion youth devising project with Carousel Players theatre. I particularly value the way RSVP postpones what RSVP director Kim Selody calls 'process-anxiety,' over time and budget pressures and production values (Selody 2006). The old 'time-talent-money' triumvirate are generally acknowledged as the weightiest pressures in the group-creation challenge.

Innovators like the international Learning Games Initiative (LGI) team assert that Rittel's morphological analysis enables a group to resist production pressures and to focus instead on a group process that leads to richness in human and product outcome. Practitioners should be alert to properties of time that easily become invisible during creation, yet are constantly affecting creative work.

How devising is a wicked problem

Collaborative theatre devising satisfies all the ten conditions Rittel uses to describe wickedness (Ruggill and McAllister 2006: 5). It requires us to work creatively with and for conflicting social forces (i.e. co-creators, producers, publics), working these group dynamics simultaneously across numerous categories of knowing, with continually shifting hierarchies and creative partnerships, sifting and sharing our values and beliefs while responding sensitively to others (Harris and Protezen 2010).

There are so very many pressures that can fragment devising groups. Often, devising leads to exhaustion, artistic dissatisfaction, and poor communication due to internal squabbles and external pressures of production. Criticism from within the group stifles inventive play; endlessly inventive play is bewildering unless some rules bring order; order and selection rules often empower leaders who then dominate discussion and goal setting. Our extrovert culture tells us that only extroverts will drive the creative process (Cain 2012), but such leadership often restricts the exploration of diverse ideas so that quieter group members disconnect, and this silences inspiration and kills collaboration.

Of all the pressures, time-and-process-anxiety is the principal, crippling fear. I mean the Murphy's Law that 'No matter how much time you have to create, two-thirds of the creative decisions are always made in the last third of the time available.' This makes us anxious. Exacerbated by capitalist values of work-time efficiency and product market-readiness, fear of 'running out of time' merges with fear of how audiences will react. As Barbara Adam says, time places a limiting condition on the ideology of will and the illusion of control (Hoffman 2009: 189). We should follow the Manual! Why are we wasting all this time? We'll never be ready by Opening! Time is money! Set goals and make a decision! Set the scene and polish it! Control! Polish! Finish!

Unfortunately, a wicked problem cannot be solved by setting goals (Conklin 2005: 5). Robert Lepage and Marie Brassard seem aware of this: they avoid a step-by-step goal setting process or 'finishing' a show, usually until it has been produced in several iterations. Given the need to define a show that is still evolving in order for media to connect devisers with potential audiences, it takes huge powers of resistance to refuse closure (Raby 1989). Refusing to pronounce a project 'finished' fits Rittel's premise that the solution to the wicked problem is never certain and cannot be objectively evaluated. Likewise, a devising team cannot select from a few options but must use all available alternatives before the project has been fully explored, and in a wicked problem, there are many contradictory alternative potential solutions. Devisers must 'collectively exercise creativity and judgment about an elegant resolution of *all* the project's priorities' until there are no alternatives left to explore (Conklin 2005: 9). LGI describes collaborative creators as used car salesmen: 'No reasonable offer refused!' (Ruggill and McAllister 2006).

This exhaustive exploration defies a product-oriented approach by requiring that the problem be reformulated at the atomic level of the team of creators themselves, so they become one with it, and reinvent it as their own. Lin Hixon says of Goat Island's exploration of Pina Bausch's style, 'I can mimic [Pina], but I can never capture her her-ness. The work's got to be completely transmigrated to be transformed into something new' (Davies 2006). Hixon echoes Oddey's conviction that truly open devising leads to transformative work that is mutually constitutive with the group's formation and all its relations, including with the world at large (1994: 2).

A wicked problem, by definition, cannot be grasped or understood, no matter how good your research, until after it has been completely solved and work stops. Jenny Hughes, Jenny Kidd and Catherine Macnamara recognize this when they speak of the need to embrace 'difficult moments of not knowing' or 'swampy lowlands' (Kershaw and Nicholson 2011: 188). Devisers avoid 'end-gaining,' as Alexander practitioners call it: planned outcomes that rigidify while codifying process (Park 1992: 119). As systems analyst Jeff Conklin puts it, a wicked problem has 'no stopping rule' or recognizable moment of completion. It is a 'one shot operation' because each wicked problem is unique to itself (Conklin 2005: 9).

Conklin observes that a common reaction when confronted with a wicked problem is to deny its wickedness and to propose a systematic approach in order to 'tame' it (Conklin 2005: 10). The 'waterfall' design process attempts to tame problems by breaking them down into categories. How often have we heard (and in my case taught), 'Gather Data; Analyse Data; Define the Problem and Set Goals; Research the Goals; Analyse and Update the Goals; Get the group to commit to the Goals; Formulate the Goals into a Solution; Polish and Produce'? Conklin says the 'waterfall' approach is the most commonly taught creative design process, but that its goal-and-outcome orientation will always be defeated by the sheer complexity of wickedness (Figure 10.1).

Devising demands inter- and intra-group collaboration at a level of creative complexity that tamer, more conventional, theatre does not. Most institutions employ a 'tough love' philosophy that requires students to learn experientially on the job after being 'dropped in at the deep end.' Students are put to work in

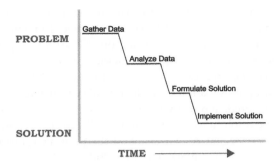

FIGURE 10.1 'Waterfall' design process.

devising groups without a framework of group dynamics or evaluative techniques. Through individualized artistic training, learning to say 'yes' in improvisation, and a brief introduction to the waterfall approach to creative design, students are expected to be good devisers.

The RSVP cycles help by making 'the creative process visible,' as Libby Worth and Helen Poynor put it (2004: 111). They allow 'opportunities for the entire group to participate,' to learn their collaborative styles, comfort zones and to reach beyond them, while 'the cyclical nature of the RSVP model emphasizes process rather than goal' (ibid.). The cycles help a collaborating team enter fully into the 'unknown' of devising at the wicked extreme of the spectrum by embracing the wicked situation and making it transparent, rather than by attempting to tame it.

How RSVP embraces wickedness to relieve the pressure of time

As many people are aware, RSVP is an acronym for the different creative mindsets that can generate a cycle of creative energies. I learned it third-hand from Robert Lepage and Marie Brassard, who learned it from Jacques Lessard, who studied with Anna Halprin. The vocabulary alters as different artists adapt RSVP for different uses, and its versatility is as impressive as its effectiveness. RSVP operates uniquely in each project that applies it.

In RSVP you cycle between four different yet mutually interdependent mindsets, hip-hopping randomly from **R**esource investigative play **(R)**, to **S**coring or arranging content materials **(S)**, to e**V**aluative analysis **(V)**, to sharing **P**erformance presentations **(P)**. The four modes of activity engage different creative intelligences that excite different strategies. Cycling between them keeps you perpetually off-balance. In wicked problem-solving, this is called 'positive disruption' (Kolko 2012), and it prevents controllers and experts from taking over. In Table 10.1, Tim Ritchey describes the General Morphological Analysis (GMA) that social planners developed for use in tackling global wicked problems such as climate change (2013: 12). But the principles can still be seen in the human scale RSVP cycles that I have put in the corresponding columns.

TABLE 10.1 Comparison of GMA and RSVP process, adapted from Tom Ritchey (2013) (adapted from Rosenhead, London School of Economics, 1996)

General Morphological Analysis	The RSVP Cycles
• Accommodate multiple alternative perspectives, functioning through group interaction rather than back-office calculations.	• Design play based on subjective Resources drawn from all group members (memory, identity, origin, experience) as well as objective Resources (materials the group chooses from art, music, objects, environment, budget, etc.).
• Engage with a number of iterative steps or phases which represent cycles of analysis and synthesis but do not aim for closure.	• Cycle through each mode in every session. Alternate modes to jump from (R) proximity and immersion in the work to (V) distance and observation, (S) organizing the material in a closed way and (P) sharing reactions to open it up through performance. Postpone scriptwriting or closure.
• Identify and define the most important dimensions of the problem complex.	• Analyse the meanings of all the materials presented. Question all assumptions in the work, separating out and labelling the power issues, cultural norms, relationship blind spots or behavioural habits that make up the different components of the problem (V).
• Explore a range of relevant values or conditions for each aspect of the problem.	• Test and explore all possible meanings via a multiplicity of scores (expressive forms, exercises, games) (V, R, S).
• Generate ownership of the problem formulation through stakeholder participation and transparency.	• Involve respondents from outside the group (P); focus on real-world impact so the group does not become insular. Filter outside feedback through group knowledge developed during the project.
• Focus on relationships between discrete alternatives rather than continuous variables.	• Decide within the group which specific material to build on (V), then continue cycling, zeroing in on content but avoiding closure.
• Facilitate a graphical (visual) representation of the problem space for the systematic, group exploration of a solution space.	• Facilitate numerous dramatic representations of the problem spaces and seek insights to build upon (S, V).
• Concentrate on possibility rather than probability.	• Problematize social clichés, stereotypes and mediatized tropes (V) and explode expectations.

LGI maintains, 'every collaboration is also an exploration of ethics, responsibility, epistemology, and ideology ... because group members are constantly forced to reevaluate their ways of seeing in order to work with one another' (Ruggill and McAllister 2006: 2). The work tends to be transformative; exit questionnaires following the Commotion project revealed that collaborators experienced what Michael Carroll describes as a 'triple loop' (2010: 15) of meta-learning about self, group and world, where attitudes, assumptions and values are explored and not just accepted from a single frame of reference. I started Commotion as a pilot project in collaboration with Kim Selody, artistic director of Carousel Players, with the goal of using RSVP to devise work with students aged 16 to 18 (seniors at two high schools in Niagara). Following the pilot and a similar program at Brock University, a Social Science and Humanities Research Council (SSHRC) grant enabled work with Carousel's subsequent artistic director Pablo Felices-Luna on a further six projects over three years (my documentary film, entitled Commotion, is available at: http://www.gyllianraby.ca). Carousel Players produced the work in their downtown St. Catharine's Theatre in Niagara and, although the RSVP production approach was replicated, the works were radically different.

The Commotion experience persuaded me that RSVP disrupts the time-forward 'arrow' of process-anxiety that governs a production plan at the macro level where there are sequential deadlines. Fear of the production schedule was calmed by the valorizing of affective rhythms that operate at the micro level described by Malcom Gladwell as a 'blink'-type spontaneity (Gladwell 2005). RSVP's focus on intuition, immediate expressivity and group experience not only distracted participants from process-anxiety, but largely replaced it.

We don't usually notice our experience of time. Barbara Adam is amazed at this, given how time is used 'to regulate, measure and control aspects of mind, body, nature and social life' (2010: 20). Drawing on the philosopher-poet Ilya Bernstein, I think that, instead of experiencing time as a steady sequence popularly imaged as 'the arrow of progress towards perfection,' RSVP participants cycle through differing scales of time (2011: 107).

RSVP diverts the time's arrows of progress and perfection

Creators experience time differently in each of the RSVP modalities and I hope my descriptions here will be intuitively familiar to most people. For example, we have all experienced the 'flight' of time as we immerse in play with the objects, images and interactions of Resource (**R**) (Figure 10.2).

The boundaries of time dissolve and flow in a legato experience. Most people remember special connections with creative sources and play practices that they learned in un-stressed periods of their lives (Drewes and Schaefer 2013: 5). Knowing that the Resource play activities can't possibly be used for a show, we laugh more, free-associate more and risk more. If collaborators realize we have happened on some interesting content and start to organize and shape it 'for the

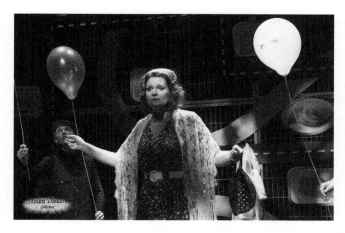

FIGURE 10.2 Danielle Wilson in *The Ash Mouth Man*, Stolen Theatre's 2017 noire comedy about ambition and eating disorder. Resource play with helium balloons shaped the devising work.

show,' it can be easy for the Resource work to segué into Scoring work; but RSVP awareness enables the group to decide whether to protect play-time or to cycle into applying scores. When we do eventually switch modalities into Scoring, the time signature of our activities changes with our mindset.

During Scoring (**S**), participants' sense of time is shaped by stepping in and out of a series of exercises, or coded notations, or sets of rules, or obstacle course shapes. Time is staccato. We experience many beginning-middle-endings, instructions, scales and dramaturgies as we struggle with the rules of the activities. Time does flow as we throw ourselves into particular exercises, but it stops when one activity ends and another begins. It is tempting and inevitable for devisers to want to stop to analyse the various arrangements of materials explored during Scoring. 'Why don't we do it again but this time improve the....' usually signals a move into an Valuaction phase where meanings are being sought and sharpened. Generally, a group can incorporate a brief hiccup of discussion into the staccato time of the activity. However, if assessments become long-winded and the activities de-rail into judgment or decision-making, the energy of the group will tip out of the staccato energy of Scoring into the allegro of Valuaction.

Valuaction, as coined by Anna Halprin, means 'the value of the action,' or 'the analysis, appreciation, feedback, value building and decision-making that accompanies the process of creation' (Poynor and Worth 2004: 112). Participants' sense of time takes on an allegro pattern with crescendos and falls; silences at the 'dredging' points of reflection; and, moments of cerebral intensity that kick in when the meanings and significances of the work are articulated. The status of participants and alliance groupings changes as agreements and disagreements escalate, and the session becomes a hot-button zone. Valuaction can be intense enough to fragment groups, so RSVP emphasizes action – *acting out* the opinions and parlaying ideas into Resources and Scores that, by changing the time signature, releases the energetic pressure. Dissent is weighed and measured, which can feel difficult, but once creators see the friction of a good Valuaction kick-start a new cycle of research and play, they grow their trust in the group's capacity to cope with diversity.

In my experience, problems with devising usually come from an over-emphasis or an under-emphasis on eValuacting. Controller team members 'at home' in the Valuaction mode often critique too soon and too much, effectively shutting down exploration. On the other hand, a group that is afraid of conflict and discord will avoid Valuaction altogether, and so won't benefit from the multiple perspectives available in the group, and won't achieve the social learning that occurs when clashing opinions are channelled into creative exercise. The allegro rhythm of intense discussion sometimes makes people feel too rattled to move into sharing/Participation activities, and it's often useful to return to the legato of Resource play before attempting to share.

Participative performance (**P**) encompasses deep listening as well as presentational sharing. This mode is empathic, comparative and comprehensive, rather than analytical: in Participative performance, we absorb the work presented and allow ourselves to be changed by the work. This usually opens a legato space with fugal echoes from the other modalities. The 'now' of the present moment becomes broader and deeper as the group expands its pool of shared images, stories, and inter- and intra-personal understandings. In Commotion, we opened the work to a forum audience of about 60 community 'friendly experts,' who gave us feedback and helped ground the project in the real world.

The Participative performance phase allows the 'slow time' of reflection and absorption (Hoffman 2009: 87). It is usually in this mode that a group realizes what we want to say in the work and develops a sense of uniqueness and its own aesthetic values. The slow time of Participation helps to process the memory that informs identity, as Eva Hoffman says in her multidisciplinary meditation on time:

> In order to make meaning of our memories (and the experiencesfrom which they flow), we need to give them our affective attention, to filter them through the scrims of our own subjectivity and absorb them into the networks of memories and selves we already are.
>
> *(Ibid.)*

Keith Johnstone articulates her point theatrically when he tells improvisers to 'walk backwards' in order to weave meanings and patterns into their narratives (1999: 116). Only by looking back at what has already gone by can we shape the steady flow of time-and-content into storied meaning, threading up the dramaturgies that turn information content into meaning.

Managers with an eye on production values and project costs are usually the greatest enemies of the slow time of in-process Performance. Sometimes, devising facilitators alert their participants to group processes by using a team management vocabulary, such as Margerison's Team Management Systems (2015). This corporate lingo can be useful in explaining relations within a devising group. The Team Management argument would assert that the deviser-group 'buys time' to develop a pool of shared images, experiences, interests and issues. Team members are forced out of their comfort zones, become better or drop out and the survivors then 'buy into the process.' In team management terms, buying in means that participants value the work they are creating more than the work they see in the world outside their group, and more than they fear failure. Buying in is thus a critical step towards 'commitment to the work,' 'owning' the material and becoming a true 'company' in the traditional sense of 'standing unified behind our product.'

This proprietary terminology flattens the temporal experience of the group into the 'arrow forward' time of a production line; it contributes to the endgaining waterfall paradigm described earlier, what is sometimes referred to as the 'storming, norming, reforming, performing' personnel relations phases. In my experience, however, the ways in which group bonding occurs are so different for every group that labelling them with a structural marker on an evolutionary timeline seems irrelevant.

I don't deny that the complete 'buy in' that celebrates any creators' fight through uncertainty and discord to stand absolutely behind their work, is common among devisers. It makes me uneasy, though, not just because of the traumatic bonding it calls for but because interpersonal power struggle encourages devisers to avoid the Valuaction that sets the creative bar high. It is devisers' passionate belief in their work that makes theatre programs give them what they want: an empty space to devise in. But as Ric Knowles has said, the space is never 'empty' (2010: 27). In the case of devising, it is a space filled with the wickedness of social assumptions waiting to colonize the unwary, unless Valuaction is understood as a necessary phase of creating.

Devising is like the wicked problem of renovating a body or a major train station while it continues to operate. The members, autonomous in their different key functions, keep radically different time, but they find a collectivity where all their priorities are met and the thing works. Students should be equipped with the ability to travel between time scales, rather than merely riding Eddington's arrow of time. The more wicked the project, the more important are the possibilities of the different creative time-zones available to us.

References

Adam, B. (2010) *Timewatch: The Social Analysis of Time*, Cambridge: Polity Press.

Bernstein, I. (2011) 'Time lines and time scales,' in Ast, O. (ed.) *Infinite Instances: Studies and Images of Time*, London: Thames and Hudson, 104–7.

Cain, S. (2012) *Quiet: Unlocking the Power of Introverts in a World that Can't Stop Talking*, New York, NY: Crown Publishing Group.

Carroll, M. (2010) 'Supervision: critical reflection for transformational learning, Part 2,' *The Clinical Supervisor*, 29: 1–19, http://www.supervisioncentre.com/docs/kv/supervision_critical_reflection_for_transformational_learning.pdf.

Conklin, J. (2005) *Dialogue Mapping: Building Shared Understanding of Wicked Problems*, Hoboken, NJ: Wiley.

Davies, G. (2006) *Creating Physical Theater: The Body in Performance*, DVD, New York: Distributed by Insight Media.

Drewes, A.A. and Schaefer, C.E. (2013) *The Therapeutic Powers of Play: 20 Core Agents of Change*, New York: Wiley.

Gladwell, M. (2005) *Blink: The Power of Thinking Without Thinking*, New York: Little, Brown.

Halprin, L. and Halprin, A. (1969) *The RSVP Cycles: Creative Processes in the Human Environment*, New York: Doubleday.

Harris, D.J. and Protzen, J.-P. (2010) *The Universe of Design: Horst Rittel's Theories of Design and Planning*, New York: Routledge.

Hoffman, E. (2009) *Time*, New York: Picador.

Johnstone, K. (1999) *Story Telling for Improvisers*, London: Routledge.

Kershaw, B. and Nicholson, H. (eds) (2011) *Research Methods in Theatre and Performance*, Edinburgh: Edinburgh University Press.

Knowles, R. (2010) *Theatre and Interculturalism*, London: Palgrave Macmillan.

Kolko, J. (2012) 'The ethics of disruptive innovation in wicked problems,' *Austin Centre for Design Faculty Student Blog*, http://www.ac4d.com/2012/04/22/the-ethics-ofdisruptive-innovation-in-wicked-problems/#sthash.5R0ytpBA.d.pdf.

Mackinnon, J. (2015) 'Personal conversation in St. Catharines, Niagara: "Devising and the Drama Department",' 7 October 2015.

Margerison, C. and McCann, D. (2015) 'Team management systems U.K.,' http://www.tmsworldwide.com/podcasts/.

Oddey, A. (1994) *Devising Theatre: A Practical and Theoretical Handbook*, New York: Routledge.

Park, G. (1992) *The Art of Changing: A New Approach to the Alexander Technique Moving towards a Freer and More Balanced Expression of the Whole Self*, Bath: Ashgrove Press.

Raby, G. (1989) Conversations during Polygraph, 1989, Arbury, Stephen (ed.), unpublished journal, 181–190.

Ritchey, T. (2013) 'Wicked problems: modelling social messes with morphological analysis,' *Acta Morphologica Generalis*, 2(1).

Ruggill, J. and McAllister, K. (2006) 'The wicked problem of collaboration,' *M/C Journal*, 9(2): 27, http://journal.media-culture.org.au/0605/07 ruggillmcallister.php.

Selody, K. (2006) Debriefing session following *Commotion* pilot production of Spin Cycle, 22 April 2006.

Wessels, A. (2012) 'Plague and paideia: sabotage in devising theatre with young people,' *RiDE: The Journal of Applied Theatre and Performance*, 17(1): 53–72.

Worth, L. and Poynor, H. (2004) *Anna Halprin*, London: Routledge.

SECTION IV

Over time

Age, duration, longevity

11

FORMATIVE TRAININGS IN CARNATIC VOCAL MUSIC

A three-way conversation through time

Tim Jones

TIM JONES (TJ): Indu, I have a memory of a story of your father and Kunjamini as young boys living in Ambalappuzha Sri Krishna temple, him training to be a temple musician, Kunjamini a *pujari* (priest). The story goes that they planted the tree that has now grown and whose many, many entwined roots and branches give cool and shade to visitors and devotees. It is near the large square podium that holds the *mizhavu*, to the left of the East Gate.[1] I love this story, the tree growing as they did, the entwined lineages of music and devotion, giving shade.

Did you tell it to me?

In 1984–1985, I was part of an intercultural theatre collaboration between Pan Project and Sopanam Theatre in Kerala, India. There I met K. R. Sivasankara Panikkar (b. 1936), Sopanam's musical director and vocal coach, and began an association lasting until his death in 2008. I spent two long study periods in Kerala singing with him. I came knowing nothing about South Indian music and sat in his small school with children aged sometimes only six or seven, learning as they learned, a beginner, a 'child voicer' in this music. I scratched the surface of the vast Carnatic repertoire and saw and loved the art forms that astonished me with their power: Sopanam, Theyyam, Sarpampattu and, of course, Kathakali.[2]

My association with *guruji* gave entry to this vibrant music, theatre and ritual arts culture. This was a time of an active, national move to promote India's performance traditions and to preserve and document arts 'heritage' on sound and video recordings. There was a theatre and film culture with auteur directors and poet playwrights, their actors training in the gesturally expressive body and vocal forms derived from Kathakali and the martial art form of Kalaripayattu. In some ways, this was also part of a 'growing' of Kerala's artistic culture, a democratizing of the rigorous training attached to these forms.

This chapter takes the form of a three-way conversation through time between three generations: *guruji*, myself and Indu (1971–), his daughter, who also taught me and the various groups I later took to Kerala.[3] In our first conversation, Indu told of how the stories and myths surrounding the composers were what first ignited her interest as a child: Tyagaraja, who wandered and spontaneously composed as he stood before the *murthi* ('form of the deity') at temples, or Muthuswami Dikshitar, whose birth was foretold by the Devi in a dream to his childless parents.[4]

INDULEKHA P. (IP): I was also very interested to listen to my father's childhood memories. He shared with me that, when he was a small child, one day he took a papaya leaf and on it made holes and started playing music. His mother noticed this, told his father, and they decided to send him, their eldest son, to learn music. His mother was also good in music. Maybe he learned from her first. The family home was at Ettumanur. There was also a guru's house and that guru had a *nadhaswaram* made of gold.[5] He started his lessons with him.

TJ: You always spoke strongly of your father teaching from within the traditional *gurukula* system, where the student (*sishya*) lives with the teacher (*guru*). I felt this at the time to be my experience; this was what I was living, albeit temporarily. I was being given a complete (very early-age!) holding environment of sound and in the full attention of a teacher. My task was to repeat, as absolutely exactly as I could, what he sang, from the pattern to the feeling and energy with which he imbued it. This format – he sings, I repeat – often continued for three hours or more. I had to bring presence to the fullness of my ability, and often, when I flagged or became muddled in the tumbling of notes, your father would only say 'you're tired,' and then we would continue.

IP: I am not confident, because I did not get any individual class from him. My father never entered me for any musical competition. Nowadays we can see if parents are very selfish in giving hard training for competitions to their children. But he was an entirely different person. In my tenth grade, I, without his permission, attended a classical music competition held by my school and I got first prize. That *kirtana* I learned from an audio cassette I heard on the loudspeakers of our temple, Charamparampu ('the place of the ash').[6] In our home we had no radio or cassette player. I showed that certificate to my father and he was very proud of that incident.

Very early I was taken by rhythm.

The music of South India is one of great rhythmic complexity and sophistication. The musician learns to keep to a rhythmic cycle of, say, 6, 7, 8, 10, 14 or more beats and, through *manodharma* ('creativity') within a formal composition, sings or plays over extended repetitions of that basic cycle. The initial training task is to keep the cycle through a mixture of hand gestures known as *mudras*, beaten out on the leg. Rhythmic cycles always end on the first beat of a cycle, so leaving a sense of openness to time's next cycle.

IP: Every summer vacation, I joined in my father's class. And singing with his students, students of all different levels, older and younger than me, I had to sit with them all until he stopped teaching. That means then a different batch arrives, so all over again!

And he was very strict. I still remember: the whole time I am making rhythm on my thigh and I feel pain there, so I beat out the rhythm with my hand on the leg of the student next to me. Suddenly, my father threw a stick at me, the stick used for making rhythm for dance, and, after that, I had to stand that full vacation outside class. Though it was painful, my father taught me a good lesson. From that moment, I learned all lessons seriously and I made efforts to remove any faults from my part. I understood his dedication. Sometimes he forgot to take his breakfast and lunch because of continuous teaching.

Every Thursday, I used to teach at Chinmaya Mission in Chittoor. Because of my strictness, there is a lot of complaining too. If they don't come regularly, I ask for reasons, very strictly. Some of them were afraid, but nowadays, when I see some of them, they tell me that I am a dedicated teacher.

TJ: I remember when Pan Project brought your father over to London to teach at a summer school (1986). Speaking no English, he would pick up and copy our speech rhythms, gradually morphing them into *konnakol* patterns of Carnatic music. I heard that the love of rhythm in Kerala derives from the sound of the thunder and monsoon rain beating on the roofs, the leaves of the trees and that beautiful red earth! You must have heard that since the day you were born!

IP: Yes, I got rich lessons in *talam*![7]

Rhythmic cycles are mastered through 'patterning,' singing sequences of notes fitting to the particular cycle, in three speeds, and at each speed in *aakaram*: every vowel. One pattern could last an hour. The physical expression of the cycle through the *mudra* mixes with the mathematical agility needed to maintain the pattern of notes, and allies with the desire to allow the 'shining' of each note, however slow, however fast the tempo.

In that extended stay of four months, there were three days towards the middle when I was singing.

Nothing more, nor less; there was only singing, with awareness of the singing of the sound not being different from the state of consciousness that was singing it. What I have called 'patterning' also reaches a point where a basic template of 'there is pattern' (patterns within patterns that evolve through breath, phrasing and expression) takes over.

On recordings from my second time training in Kerala (1988–1989), there is a demonstration of teaching strategies by Indu's father. He was showing me four stages of his approach with students: first kindly, a playful coaxing; then a firmer presence asking for engagement; then a stern demand for presence; and finally, force that could include an explosive 'get out of my sight!' All through sung sound, gesture and *abhinaya* ('aesthetic expression of emotion'). I saw the various stages of this in action with students of all ages, professional singers and actors as well as children sometimes only six or seven years old.

On another recording, he sings a song. 'Sarasa sama dana,' the composition by Tyagaraja. It sings of the four strategies, *sama-dana-bheda-danda*, used artfully by Rama in dealing with the demon Ravana within the Hindu epic, *The Ramayana*:

> Ravana [...] did not know you are an artful expert of
> timely, friendly persuasion, wise gifting
> dividing to conquer, and lastly, use of force.
>
> *(Jackson 1991: 319)*

What I had taken to be a personal teaching strategy emerged, then, directly from *within* musical and spiritual traditions as sound, story, singing, gesture and feeling.

IP: With his friend who was a great dance master, Natuvar Paramasivam, my father started a new school for music and dance named Sauparnika.[8] Sauparnika is a name of the sacred river at Mookambika. My father was a great devotee of Mookambika. In that school, I restarted music from him.

At one time, Tulasi, his student, visited my home to see my father. She stayed for one day and she sang and my mother sang with her. The carpenter doing renovations was my father's friend. He asked why I was not being sent to music college. My father refused.

TJ: Was that the same Tulasi your father taught?

IP: Yes. He had just begun teaching at Ambalappuzha. This small girl would stand at the window watching and listening in to the class: he noticed it. One day, as he walked unknowingly by her house, he heard a young girl's voice singing. He called the child's mother and asked her to send the child to attend class. The child had lost her father and, the family being very poor, her mother says: 'we can't pay fees.' My father assured her there was no need to pay the fees, just to send her daughter for music lessons. Tulasi started learning from him and became a famous Carnatic musician.

I asked Tulasi to get an application form from Tripunithura College where she was teaching. I fixed in my mind, 'I learn music only, I don't take any other.' A big fight happened with me refusing to take food, crying until finally my father agreed. The day before my interview, I went to Tulasi's home. I sang 'Bhairavi ada tala varnam' (the oldest known *varnam* or extended teaching song) that I learned from my father's class.[9] Then, on the day of the interview, in the early morning, I went to Poornathrayeesa Temple and it was my great experience. I became a big devotee of Poornathrayeesa god.[10] It was my first time in this temple. I loved this place and I wanted to live there. This was more than 26 years ago, and now I live in this place with my family under the blessings of this god.

At that time, after my studies, I moved back to Alleppey and started music classes there. I got small children and two college students too. I too am very strict. I never entertained my students singing from notation. I told them to look at the teacher's face and sing. Very strict, like my father!

I was born at a time when my father was performing at Mullakkal Temple in Ambalappuzha, a temple renowned for being accessible to devotees from all castes and religions. I try to teach in that spirit now, teaching many different people. I teach one child with autism. I observed that child, and I saw that there is no coordination of the eyes to his attention. I remembered my father's words, 'look to the teacher's eye in learning.' So, every time, I touch his hand and say: 'look at my eyes, you can see, there at my eyes.' He has started looking at me and a big change happens in him. I also teach children with disabilities. They're very interested in learning music. Music learning will develop children's concentration, confidence, memory. It also helps their vocabulary. Most of the students like Western music, and I start to teach that too. I give them voice training. Now most of them are very good in singing, some of them love to sing Indian songs!

TJ: And I teach Indian songs here in England!

IP: I want to tell you one more thing. Tripunithura is a royal city with many chances to meet with great artists. There is a Temple festival time that attracts many concerts by legends. I was very interested in Madurai T.N. Seshagopalan's style of singing.[11] His technique is like my father's. I fixed in my mind that I would like to study from him. A concert was arranged for him at Ambalappuzha near our home. I asked my father: 'I want to talk with him and I would like to touch his feet for blessing.' I went to the temple with my brother Ani and father. My father was very busy. He knows Seshagopalan personally. I did not get a chance for blessing. My father would not help me in this. I was very sad. I cried and left the place saying that Lord Krishna cheated me. We reached Alleppey by train. The railway station was empty. My brother went for tea. It was very early in the morning, and suddenly I saw Seshagopalan very near to me and he smiled. With a big cry, I touched his feet for blessing, and we talked a lot, and soon after, I started my studies with him.

This marks the beginning of another cycle in Indu's narrative of Carnatic voice training: Sivasankara (and Kunjamini) as young trainees at the temple; Indu as a child, training in her father's class, then with Seshagopalan; Tulasi, a 'small girl' accessing voice lessons through Sivasankara's invitation, helping Indu apply for training; Indu now training young, diverse Carnatic voicers, strict as her father in the teaching of rhythm. And myself, a novice trainee among children trainees in the late 1980s, a 'child' in training, now teaching voice and song from the source of that immersion. These cycles of embodied pedagogy call to mind the 'patterning' of metric structures, of the *talam*: formally repeated but open-ended, inviting creativity and life.

In highlighting this generational timeline, this essay suggests that there might be a generational timeline *of the training*, the training seeding itself (not unlike the tree planted by Sivasankara), renewing itself in ways that are not simply of the individual and separate journeys from novice to mature performer. We can be mindful of the many aspects of training, the complexity and strata of its make-up and the particulars of what each trainee brings to, and absorbs for, their own development of the tradition. So, the growth and evolution is nurtured by the sympathies of those living with and within rather than shaped by complicity in the preservation of a preexisting edifice.

In each generational cycle, might there be a (re)new(ed) 'young adulthood' of the training itself? Certainly, if I look at my own experience and reflect on my artistic practice, I feel both lines of growth from my training and see what was open in me to receive it – and I also see this in Indu's narrative. Some things stare me in the face: a current practice, 'a choreography of speaking singing' seems to be my unwitting branch, 30 years later, of Sivasankara's own research and interest in the connection of *Angikabhinayam* ('body language') with *Vachikabhinayam* ('dialogue delivery') developed through his 'theatre music.' I would like to acknowledge his research, creativity and openness in this.

Indu's narrative brings its own complexity, revealing a multifaceted landscape of different experiences of training: informal/everyday, formal, teaching as *retraining*. Her biographical reflections invite us to embrace formative training as woven into a more cyclical, layered, porous and expansive conceptualization of time lived in and through training. In it, we encounter varied notions of time, strata if you will: time as it is lived and remembered; time in the long game of tradition, in its musical, rhythmical sense; and time in its immediate, culturally understood, sense of cycles, the seasons and their festivals, the daily rituals at the temple, and of the 432,000 years of the Kali Yuga (the Age of Conflicts, part of the four ages of the world that themselves form a cyclical whole lasting 4,290,000 years). And we encounter story-time, different experiences of recurrence and of wishes seeded long ago coming to fruition in unexpected ways and in a fullness of time.

Notes

1 The *mizhavu* is a percussion instrument accompanying the dance drama form Koodiyattam.
2 Sopanam ('temple steps') is a form of storytelling, the sung recitation of 'Gita Govinda,' a 12th-century poem by Jayadeva. Theyyam is a ritual dance drama from North Kerala, often telling the story of the goddess Bhadrakali and the demon Darikan. Sarpampattu is a ritual to the *naga* ('snake deities'), involving ritual powder drawing and trance possession of the female dancers.
3 Indu now teaches at TIPS (The Indian Public School), Kochi.
4 The Trinity, Dikshitar (1775–1835), Tyagaraja (1767–1847) and Syama Shastri (1762–1827), are still the bedrock of the classical tradition (arguably 'classical' in a move to establish an existing tradition as 'classical' after the Western model; see Weidman 2006).
5 A double-reed hardwood wind instrument often used at weddings and temple rituals.

6 *Kirtana* is a song form.
7 *Talam* is rhythmic cycle.
8 Sauparnika opened in 1979.
9 *Bhairavi* is the *ragam* ('melody form'), *ada* is the *talam* and *varnam* is the song form.
10 Lord Vishnu, who, at Poornathrayeesa sits under the shade of the five royal hoods of the divine serpent, Ananthan, whose folded body itself acts as the throne for the God.
11 Seshagopalan (1948–) is a renowned Carnatic vocalist.

References

Jackson, W.J. (1991) *Tyagaraja: Life and Lyrics*, Oxford: Oxford University Press.
Weidman, A.J. (2006) *Singing the Classical, Voicing the Modern: The Postcolonial Politics of Music in South India*, Durham, NC: Duke University Press.

12

CHANGE, CONTINUITY AND REPETITION

Married to the Balinese mask

Tiffany Strawson

This chapter situates traditional training for *topeng*, the Balinese Masked–Dance drama within culturally specific temporalities which nuance the experience of performer training in Bali. Using David E. R. George's statement as a point of departure, discussion concerns how a specific training followed in the traditional way, in this case *topeng*, can be considered as part of wider, intercultural performer training.

> All theories of time have to confront a basic philosophical problem, one as much logical as empirical; the problem of continuity and change. They form a classic binary; everything changes, but to be recognized as the thing which changed, something – in everything – must continue. You can only have change if there is continuity and vice versa.
>
> *(George 1999: 44)*

Whilst offering insight into traditional practices and cultural constructions of time, the focus is on the encounter between different temporalities in terms of traditional and intercultural practitioners of the *topeng* genre. The intercultural practitioners that I am interested in are women who take on the traditional roles of men, as *topeng* is traditionally and predominantly a male genre. Gender issues aside,[1] of interest in this chapter, is the question of how to maintain a practice as one becomes less physically able to deliver the virtuosity of youth and what is traded or exchanged as the performer acquires an embodied wisdom.

Here, the lens of 'new' interculturalism is of value as a critical framework in that it theoretically embraces an 'embodied corporeal language with a conscious rejection of text [and] a sense of auto-ethnography and real-life experience, in–betweeness be that of nations, disciplines, culture; a disruption of the concept of othering' (Mitra 2015: 29). Performers address the longevity of their practice and their aging bodies and discuss how their attitudes continue to change with age. The dialogue offered between my own praxis, the perspectives of other intercultural practitioners and Balinese performers contextualize this analysis. The relationship between virtuosity and temporality is complex. How might the convergence of training, performing, teaching and individually packaged relationships referred to as 'marriage' serve the intercultural performer and/or the Balinese maestro in terms of virtuosity? As Balinese dancer Ni Made Pujawati remarks, 'virtuosity grows over time; teaching, performing, it gives you better confidence in characterisation' (2014) and enables the performer to embody, understand, play and enable a genuine meeting place with the mask.

The focus is on training; however, this training is significantly linked to performance in Bali. It is important to define the conditions of traditional training that apply and to contextualize this within the framework of change, development, continuity all of which produce a unique Balinese sense of temporality. What is apparent within this training is how notions of time create a relationship between the performer and the mask, that is a dynamic described as a 'marriage' and how the experience of training is aligned to performing and teaching. Grounding experiences of traditional training, within the idea of change and continuity, this chapter explores the individual experiences of an aging body within the context of a training system that embraces repetition and endurance. This balance between micro and macro exposes, on the one hand, a maturity and experience akin to the challenges of a deep training and, on the other, a naivety or lack of experience in view of the lifetime commitment necessary. For Murray, a deep training is 'a lifelong practice, an enduring unfolding, a practice of embodied critical reflection, a praxis of theory and action, of head and hand, of thought and deed' (Murray 2015: 53). In addition, other qualities of 'depth' in the context of *topeng* training include: long-standing in terms of time, duration and that which is achieved whilst in training takes time to settle in the body, knowledge which is transferable and applicable in other contexts (rather than knowledge that is finite) and finally, a vertical dissemination of knowledge from master to student where the 'hand-in-hand chain is itself symbolic of the continuity of practice and the experience of knowledge transfer' (Matthews 2014: 35).

Situating traditional training

In the traditional style of Balinese training, there is a commitment to *kebalian* meaning 'Balinese-ness' and this is bound up in *adat* (custom) and *agama* (religion) which, in *topeng*, includes spiritual worship, ceremonial offering, sacrifice and prayer. Far beyond a simple technical training, issues such as acceptable behaviour, social conduct, education and community service are among those aspects that are taught through the culturally established phenomenon of dance training and performance education (Strawson 2014: 293).

Once a basic choreography is learnt, the teacher drills the student in a military fashion until the dance is *masuk* (inside). This corresponds to Clarke's suggestion that in Asian traditions, the participant copies the 'parent' teacher by rote and imitation (Clarke 2009: 27). It is then the responsibility of the student to refine, practise and observe as much as possible and develop one's *stil sendiri* (meaning 'individual style'). Whilst this is encouraged, the student initially adopts the style of the master dancer; the teacher who physically manipulates the student's body and shapes 'him' like moulding clay. In Bali, there is a greater conscious acknowledgement for tradition than non-Balinese are familiar with and this conventionally manifests as respect for age and wisdom (Strawson 2014: 299). If one chooses to train one-to-one with a *guru*, one is embarking on a special mentor/mentee relationship. In the Balinese tradition, teachers, both male and female, often refer to their students as *anak anak*, meaning children, and this demonstrates the relationship between student and teacher. To extend the metaphor, children leave the nest but have a sense of belonging and rootedness; so the *topeng* student is expected to develop his *stil sendiri* but always give credit to the lineage of the teacher.

Training as/in performance

In Bali, there is recognition that the stage is a training ground. Performing is an inherent part of the learning process. Pujawati believes that 'the ultimate and important thing is to perform and get feedback and do it all again' (Pujawati 2011). It is understood that through time and repetition, students repeat the version of the dance instilled by their teacher until they can adapt, improvise and hold the stage on their own merit. In this environment, the performer gets to test what they have learned as they develop their relationship with their mask and thus traditional *topeng* training finds its own understanding of temporality. Traditionally, there is more opportunity to develop one's potential with a particular mask, due to the number of opportunities to perform. This could be three performances a day, several times a week. Performing the same mask repeatedly, at different times of day, in various conditions all influence the growth and development of the performance throughout a lifetime. Understanding training as/in performance is useful as this approach can be viewed 'under both rubrics (as well as their blurring)' (Parker–Starbuck and Mock 2011: 2010).[2]

Situating 'age on the Balinese stage' and notions of legacy

In Balinese topeng, one of the most popular characters for audiences is *topeng tua*, the old man mask. He represents the Autumn and Winter of life and is a comical figure (Figure 12.1).

As well as representations of age, in Bali, it is common to see senior performers dancing in ceremonial performances, on professional 'arts' circuits and festivals and in tourist shows; all of which are approached with exactly the same degree of professionalism. For example, Pak Djimat who is regarded as a professional dance maestro and particularly established in the role of *topeng dalam* (meaning the

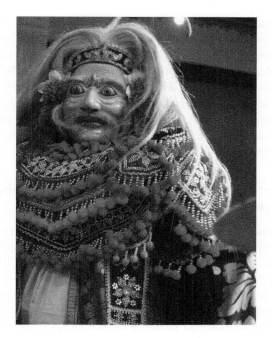

FIGURE 12.1 Sixty-four-year-old Ida Bagus Alit dances *topeng tua* in Lod Tunduh, 2006. Photo: the author.

'king' mask) performs weekly in front of tourist audiences, at the Arma Museum with a *topeng* show that features both himself, his son and his students.

Another example of senior performers and the performances that have made them famous, was in Peliatan in March 2012, at the Open Stage *Ancak Saji*, where there was a dance event called 'Spirit of Raka Rasmi' to celebrate seventy-three-year-old maestro performer Ibu Raka (Gusti Ayu Raka Rasmi). She is famous for the dance genre known as *Oleg Tamulilingan*. The performance was accompanied by Gunung Sari, the group that brought Gusti Ayu Raka to international acclaim in 1952. The performance featured Ibu Raka, and like Djimat's *topeng* show, included performances by all the dancers under her tutelage. Consistent with the notion that performing, training and teaching converge in Bali, this event included a dance workshop facilitated by Ibu Raka for all pupils. The intention was to preserve the choreography of the dance form *Oleg Tamulilingan* in the Peliatan Style and pass on her 'spirit' or what is regarded in Bali as *taksu*, which broadly means the convergence of art and spirit or 'divine charisma' (Dibia and Ballinger 2004: 11), to the following generations. At this event, Ibu Raka's daughter A. A. Istri Wirati, and granddaughter all performed parts of the same dance within a sequence. Dance ethnographer, traditional dancer, intercultural performer and long-term resident of Bali, Rucina Ballinger explained that younger generations of the same family perform the more physically exerting choreography and that this convention is becoming common (Ballinger 2016).

The reasons, she explains are twofold; it not only enables senior maestro performers to perform in dances that they themselves, through their energy and virtuosity, have become synonymous with, but also allows dance styles as well as the dancers themselves to tangibly demonstrate a sense of lineage (Ballinger 2016). It is very typical to train your own children and as mentioned previously, a teacher's student is their adopted 'child.' In both this example and the one of Djimat, there is acknowledgement that one's legacy may be expanded during one's lifetime and that a dancer's lineage, and more significantly the dance itself, is extended in and beyond one's lifetime.

Obstacles and challenges within my own *topeng* training; a brief over view

For any performer, a training regime must be balanced, devised on high ambition, practically sustainable and time managed. It is difficult for the non-Balinese trainee/performer to maintain such immersion into traditional training unless they live in Bali. During my years there, as well as the joys and rewards of training, I experienced frustration with the *topeng* choreography and the 'embodiment' of the mask for a variety of reasons. This relevant sense of auto-ethnography that offers a rationale for this research and these critical observations are relevant to all non-Balinese dancers. First, as part of the tactile 'moulding clay' dynamic, my teacher would attempt to bend back my fingers to reach my forearm. In fairness, this is how children are trained; it is *tradisi* but without the agility of youth, I realized that I was following a training regime designed for a nubile, pre-teen boy body. With a late starting female body, one can accept new challenges, however, one must also accept one's limitations. Second, although I could technically 'do it' and could theoretically appreciate the qualities of energy as articulated by the Balinese religion; 'understanding does not lead to embodied knowledge' (Turner 2011: 70). As a non-Balinese, it is difficult to realize 'full' embodiment as defined by Balinese levels of accomplishment.[3] This is pertinent in terms of embodiment, characterization and what it means to harness the 'much contested term' (Murray 2015: 46, 50–51); 'energy' in order to bring the mask to life.

Embodiment of the mask

Youth aside, there was still hope as I continued to develop my relationship with the mask through repeated activity (training and performing) gradually understanding that, as I Madé Sija asserts:

> Anyone can learn how to dance, that is *ngigel*, but this is not enough; it is superficial, it's just dance movements. What is important instead is *mesolah*, to characterise.
>
> *(Sija quoted by Palermo 2009)*

What is meant by characterization is to bring the mask to 'life'; one must study and understand the mask in its fullest capacity and this has to do with cultural history, identity, location and sense of what constitutes 'Balinese-ness.' All of which, in the Balinese context, constitute a sense of 'energy.' As Turner claims:

> (T)he notion of embodiment is a term which in Bali encompasses a spiritual element whereby the performer opens themselves to the gods who can empower them and give them divine inspiration to perform more effectively.
>
> *(2011: 70)*

Attempting to penetrate this culturally specific sense of spirituality is problematic terrain; one might, with maturity and insight, achieve a meeting place between two-world views but this is a hybrid state. Openness, flexibility and plurality may be general cultural characteristics of a more generalized Indonesian culture, but one's ability to enact any of these qualities is entirely individual. Therefore, practical approaches must consider under what timely conditions and circumstances a process of training and new 'embodied corporeal language[s]' (Mitra 2015: 29) can be developed to explore the embodiment of the mask both in and outside of Bali.

Here, the theoretical approach of 'new interculturalism' helps in the consideration of time and temporality across cultures within training. As well as including auto-ethnography as one of its features, Mitra suggests that there is a 'perpetual identification with a state of in-betweeness; between cultures, between nations, between disciplines and between the different versions of ... self, with a recognition that many other selves and many others co-exist' (2015: 29). The idea of 'in-betweeness' is bound up with notions of mobility, politics and power and it should be pointed out that the way in which these are constructed/ experienced, is particular and specific to each intercultural practice. This research has embraced 'in-betweeness' by engaging with all that entanglement; there is an attempt to disrupt binaries between East/West, male/female, youth/age, mask-maker/performer, Bali/England and by working between the disciplines of dance/drama. Whilst being 'in-between' there is always the unknown, however one's focus can also sharpen, and tune into a new set of ideas and knowledge. Within my practice, I can exchange any discomfort of being in-between with a growing confidence; an intercultural practice can occupy all of these positions equally and all positions become changeable, plural and temporal.

On a more pragmatic level, initial dance training involves how to physically emphasize different energies: the *keras* and *halus* gestures representing the hard, stiff or powerful movements and respectively those that are softer and refined. A balance between the two is the aim. Combined and integrated into these qualities are *idep* (thought), *bayu* (energy or power manifested in wind or breath) and *sabda* (voice) are often referred to as the Three Ways of Communicating or *tigajnana* (Hobart 2003: 213–14) with the holy trinity of gods Brahma, Vishnu (known in Bali as Wisnu) and Shiva (known in Bali as Siwa). This is achieved by the *pusat nabhi, the* place from where breath emerges, centrally located in the body. What is explicit is that breath is seen as an internal balancing mechanism between various poles of opposition; micro/macro, inhale/exhale, feminine/ masculine and that these poles are reflected physically in the *agem*, which are the basic standing positions forming balance through asymmetry, documented by Barba and Saravese (2006: 32–51). These energies are reflected in the choreographic movements, for example, the strong and swift movement known as '*ansel*' which represents the fiery power Brahma; '*nayog*' which is a balanced pushing, flowing movement represents Siwa; and '*ngikal*' which shows the wave-like, watery quality of Wisnu.

Whilst this training spans cultural, social and spiritual terrains, physical training is paramount in almost all performer training and therefore seeking physical comfort in a gesture is important. Previously, I had never had reason to dance with my elbows above my shoulder, with my hand palm facing the sky. Seeking comfort in a gesture demands change of position when it is no longer comfortable, if the dance is to be continued. Being 'in dialogue' with the choreography means that rather than enduring pain, finding easefulness is possible by breathing into the *agem*, so that with each inhalation one can actively visualize the (dis)comfort, stop – pause – change and reassess as necessary. In this sense, a performer can playfully engage in cultural practices that facilitate and maintain appropriate, relational responses. Pujawati explains that

> Although my knees hurt, because I continue, I remember things and now I can relax, find comfort. We train kids to bend their knees, but older people are able to characterise.
>
> *(2014)*

In this discussion of comfort, there is a paradox because Balinese dance is by nature difficult and virtuosity is the aim. Therefore, comfort is never to be replaced or confused by making the gesture 'easy'. However, easefulness can be sought through comfort so that the dance ceases to be painful. Seeking comfort during training may compromise one's gestural or expressive potential technically in performance, but it does promote actual enjoyment and expression of the choreography, which in turn expels delight in the dance. Performers experience on occasion what Fraleigh calls 'intrinsic dance' which she describes as a state of 'pleasure we feel in our bodies when we are in our own flow of being, moving for the dance and not to please others' (2000: 58). Enjoyment and delight, is closer to the higher qualities of ceremonial performance as described by the various Balinese levels of attainment. Whilst these qualities in no way replicate *taksu*, which is perceived by the audience, not the performer, they do embody the active service and commitment that the Balinese *topeng* performer may experience.

This simple change in perspective of developing enjoyment and delight through comfort is invested with a deeper sense of longevity and awareness of the mask. There is a renewed interest into the potential 'life force' of one's own, aging body and a discovery that enables one to develop a closer and more accepting relationship to one's body; where the mask and the body move together with reciprocity. Scholar and *topeng* dancer Margaret Coldiron suggests, 'the technique has to be there, but ultimately it is about the distribution of energy in the body' (2013) and practitioners of Balinese dance agree that what is important is that the use of energy (however that may be harnessed either through traditional approaches or through more nuances, personal adaptations of embodied discourses) significantly enables the performer to embody the mask and to bring it to 'life.'

A traditional Balinese performer's relationship to their mask

Balinese performers have the 'luxury of time' (Pujawati 2011). The implication is that as a performer, one can develop a relationship to that role/mask over many years. For this reason, the relationship between performer and mask, considered far more than an inanimate object, is often referred to as a 'marriage.' By that, it is understood as not only an unending bond, but also a relationship imbued with personal and cultural commitment that is socially shared and appreciated through ceremonial performance. A temple ceremony offers a unique opportunity for performers to develop their mask relationship and thus traditional *topeng* training finds its own understanding of temporality which, once committed, is a 'forever' dynamic and considered an entwined, 'spiritual' connection that is deeply rooted in a sense of personal and cultural lineage. Like any long-term committed relationship, there are rewards, challenges and problems. One of the few common elements in the discourse on mask characterization is that to bring the mask alive, the performer has to be 'one with the mask' and preferably united through a marriage ritual called *puspati*. Most performers would not allow another to use their personal mask, ceremonial masked storyteller Ida Bagus Alit jokes and says this would be 'like sharing his wife – never!' (2003).

A non-Balinese 'marriage' considered within a broader practice

In Bali, a dancer's relationship with the mask, however theoretically understood, is a challenge for the non-Balinese performer of *topeng* to fully embrace, negotiate and live by as it is deeply rooted in complex and culturally specific traditions. Any 'marriage' is personal whatever the culture, and any relationship is shaped by individual life experience, culture and society. Although many cultures share a heavy reliance on traditional expectations, outside of Bali, potentially, the notion, definition and cultural expectation of 'marriage' is more open to a flexible interpretation. Coldiron asserts that 'as I have gradually discovered, you really have to be *kawin dengan topeng* ("married with the mask")' (2014). Without a culturally embodied sense of religion, interwoven lineages and blood lines, a non-Balinese understanding of marriage is different to any Balinese understanding, so this statement needs some further unpacking. Coldiron remarked

> I have a very great sense of responsibility to the mask; masks that become inhabited, they take on a life of their own the more they are used … the more they are worn, the better they get, it's like magic.
>
> *(2016)*

Another view is expressed by scholar and *topeng* performer Carmencita Palermo who suggests that her mask relationship benefits from the combination of absence and intensity:

> After an interruption in training, after a break away from the mask, there is an improvement away from the mask, people noticed it … There are also times when I am never separated from my mask. Body, mind, mask, is that what the Balinese call a marriage?
>
> *(2016)*

Evidently, there is no fixed way for the non-Balinese performer's union with the mask to manifest, yet a marriage is what many intercultural performers define their mask relationship to be and this is based on what works for them individually. As the case of Palermo suggests, who is *kawin dengan topeng*, this relationship through absence and intensity, is no less committed, devoted and invested than any other performer.

Without the same culturally specific understanding of the mask that a Balinese performer may have, perhaps a non-Balinese relationship with a Balinese mask could be simplistically described as a marriage to the 'performer within oneself.' However, this simplification does not quite do justice to the experienced non-Balinese performer's deep understanding of Balinese culture, to the nuances of the mask and how to fully embody it. 'Marriage' becomes a metaphor for the complex and committed relationship the non-Balinese performer has, with one's very personal and intercultural performance practice where specifically, the mask becomes a united 'other,' is one-in-the-same and co-lives the performer's lifetime of training/performing.

The relationship between training and teaching

In Bali, it is culturally understood that as a performer ages, there is a propensity to start teaching. In all manners of practice, both in a traditional Balinese and intercultural non-Balinese settings,[4] teaching can vitally contribute to a sense of training, progression and professional development for the aging performer. In Bali, there is a cultural understanding of fluctuating place-time-circumstances, *desa-kala-patra*, and this conflation of place-time-circumstance can offer insight into the predominant 'younger-older' continuum with 'trainee-performer/teacher' and conflates the younger-older binary in interesting ways. This culturally specific view of the world has significant implications for both the traditional/Balinese performer and the intercultural, non-Balinese performer of *topeng*, which are relevant to issues pertaining to temporality. It offers a potentially more cyclically invested view of the approach necessary in training and performing. As was suggested earlier in the case of Ibu Raka, teaching is a vital element of her practice and legacy. Here training-teaching works in relation to the theme of time in a way that corresponds with the experiences of intercultural performers Ballinger, Coldiron and Palermo, all of whom, like myself, have experienced pain and injury whilst embracing the fact that they need to continue and develop their practice. Coldiron claims that 'teaching made me improve my technique, as you have to demonstrate in the right way' (Coldiron 2014). Palermo asserts:

> I am working more now than I was five years ago, and training depends on your life-style, what you do and when you can do it. I train differently now than when I did twenty-five years ago, of course. Now I teach a lot. I am going over, over and over the basic technique for my students and that is what I teach and that's how I do my basic training. It adds another quality to how you use your body.
>
> *(2016)*

Interestingly, Palermo acknowledges that she is 'growing in beauty while training as a teacher' (2016). This is culturally significant, as in the Balinese language, there is no word for dancer, other than *pragina* 'someone who beautifies' (Dibia and Ballinger 2004: 8). It appears in the example of these intercultural practitioners that attention to their mask relationship/'marriage,' has become slowly embedded with culturally specific Balinese precepts. These include a distinct passion for teaching, sharing, and that this dissemination cyclically feeds into the training that their bodies enable and allow them to do and need as regular basic training. The role of the teacher in Bali is highly esteemed, as was earlier discussed in the descriptions of traditional training. Ballinger asserts:

> The person who is teaching is the receptacle of knowledge which is so important in traditional oral culture. I love teaching and seeing the work manifest, there's a pride to it, not in an egotistical way, but I genuinely feel like I am a conduit of passing on something precious.
>
> *(2014)*

Through this recognition of 'passing on something precious,' there is the idea of passing something down through younger generations, and simultaneously across, through students and audiences new to this genre.

Negotiating cultural difference takes time. The implication of any temporality, where the role of energy to bring the mask to 'life' relies on the acquisition of embodied knowledge, is deeply invested with notions of change, continuity and repetition. As the body ages and responds to the passing of the years, the relationship, the 'marriage' with the mask, also resonates with a different sense of time.

Rarely do intercultural performers start training in their chosen form in their youth and more often, one adopts a performance culture other than one's 'own' later in life. In this chapter, what these *topeng* performers share is understanding, knowledge and awareness of the mask developed through deep training, cultural curiosity from both inside and outside perspectives, embodied through cultural absorption, acceptance of age and ability, settled through the experiences of injury, as well as repeated successes and failure in these attempts. All of which in turn, and in/through time, develop a wisdom and experience that allows the genre to redefine notions of virtuosity.

Notes

1 For more reading on gender and Balinese performance, see Ballinger (2005), Diamond (2008), Dibia (1990), Dibia and Ballinger (2004), Emigh (1996), Palermo (2009) and Ross (2005). For more reading on gender, Western women, topeng and interculturalism, see Coldiron et al. (2015).
2 On one occasion in Bali, I had two teachers, which does not follow the traditional apprenticeship (Strawson 2014). Both teachers were offended that I had not solely chosen them. Consequently, I was not invited to accompany either teacher to ceremonies; these revoked opportunities to dance led me to appreciate the inseparable dynamic between training, performance and tradition. They cannot exist in isolation.
3 The ultimate performance level is *Wibawa*, a term that translates as having spiritual aura, 'internal power/values' (Rubin and Sedana 2007: 125).
4 I appreciate that culture and tradition cannot be so neatly divided or generalized. There are Balinese performers working in contemporary forms, and non-Balinese performers working within traditional mediums and both these combinations could be considered intercultural.

References

Ballinger, R. (2005) 'Woman power,' in *Inside Indonesia*, 83, (July–September), 7–8.
———— (2016) Interview with T. Strawson, UK.
Barba, E. and Savarese, N. (2006) *A Dictionary of Theatre Anthropology: The Secret Art of the Performer*, Oxon: Routledge.
Clarke, A. (2009) 'Family roles and paternal/maternal genealogies within and between psychophysical performer trainings and their documentation,' *Platform: Staging Gender(s)*, 4(1): 25–43.
Coldiron, M. (2013) 'Being a Woman Being a Man: Gender and Balinese Performance' conference paper in Women in Asia conference, *13th/14th September*, Lincoln, UK: Lincoln University.
———— (2014, 17 March) 'Re; Our Topeng paper ATJ,' email message to T. Strawson, UK.
———— (2016) Interview with T. Strawson, UK.
Coldiron, M., Palermo, C. and Strawson, T. (2015) 'Women in Balinese *Topeng*: voices, reflections and interactions,' *Asian Theatre Journal*, 32(2): 464–92.
Diamond, C. (2008) 'Fire in the banana's belly: Bali's female performers essay the masculine arts,' *Asian Theatre Journal*, 25(2): 231–71.
Dibia, I.W. (1990) 'The symbols of gender in Balinese dance,' *UCLA Journal of Dance Ethnography*, 12: 10–12.

Dibia, I.W. and Ballinger, R. (2004) *Balinese Dance, Drama and Music*, Singapore: Periplus Editions.

Emigh, J. (1996) *Masked Performance, the Play of Self and Other in Ritual and Theatre*, Pennsylvania, PA: University of Pennsylvania Press.

Fraleigh, S. (2000) 'Consciousness matters,' *Dance Research Journal*, 32(1): 54–62.

George, D.E.R. (1999) *Buddhism as/in Performance*, New Delhi: D. K. Printworld (P) Ltd.

Hobart, A. (2003) *Healing Performances of Bali, Between Darkness and Light*, New York and Oxford: Berghahn Books.

Ida Bagus Alit. (2003) Interview with T. Strawson, transcript by Made Yudiana. Ubud, Bali.

Matthews, J. (2014) *Anatomy of Performance Training*, London: Bloomsbury Methuen.

Mitra, R. (2015) *Akhram Khan: Dancing New Interculturalism*, London and New York: Palgrave Macmillan.

Murray, S. (2015) 'Keywords in performer training,' *Theatre, Dance and Performance Training*, 6(1): 46–58.

Palermo, C. (2009). '"*Anak mula keto*" "It was always thus": women making progress, encountering limits in characterising the masks in balinese masked dance-drama,' *Intersections: Gender and Sexuality in Asia and the Pacific*. [Online], Issue 19, February. http://intersections.anu.edu.au/issue19/palermo.htm (Accessed 12 January 2015).

———— (2016) Interview with T. Strawson, UK.

Parker-Starbuck, J. and Mock, R. (2011) 'Researching the body in/as performance,' in Kershaw, B. and Nicholson, H. (eds) *Research Methods in Theatre and Performance*, Edinburgh: Edinburgh University Press, 210–35.

Pujawati, N.M. (2011, 2014) Interviews with T. Strawson, Plymouth, UK.

Ross, L.M. (2005) 'Mask, gender, and performance in Indonesia: an interview with Didik Nini Thowok,' *Asian Theatre Journal*, 22(2): 214–26.

Rubin, L. and Sedana, I.N. (2007) *Performance in Bali*. London and New York: Routledge.

Strawson, T. (2014) 'Dance training in Bali: intercultural and globalised encounters,' *Theatre Dance Performance Training*, 5(3): 291–303.

Turner, J. (2011) 'Embodiment, Balinese dance theatre, and the ethnographer's predicament,' *Performance and Spirituality*, 2(1) (Spring): 60–84.

13

THE FEELING OF TIME

Jennifer Jackson

Aged 40, I went to university. It was time to reflect. After 22 years as a professional ballet dancer, choreographer and co-director of a small ballet company,
I had questions about the art of dance, but little time to ponder. Many colleagues
who were curious about dance had found fruitful territory for exploration and
discovery in academia and contemporary dance forms, and I half expected that
my passion for ballet would crumble in the face of feminist critiques of its forms
and practices. However, my year of intense theoretical study led me back to ballet and forwards into deeper conversations and new ways of seeing. It taught me
that the mind could hold apparently paradoxical ideas in the same space. I saw
that dancing, being in the body/mind as a dancer, was a way of resolving and
harmonizing different ideas. I could be a feminist *and* a ballet dancer. But for all
the theory and thinking that these studies had seeded, there was something dead
at the heart of my practice. It was time for action – back into the studio, back
into class. A new colleague, Patrick Wood[1] introduced me to his teacher, Roger
Tully, and 22 years on, I am still dancing.[2]

Tully's studio is an unusual environment for training in ballet. His concept, 'that
you have the ideal body for your own dance' (Jackson: 2005), offered a radically
different approach to practice.[3] On more subtle levels, his class opened a fresh way
of experiencing time in training that has proved grounding *and* liberating. Dance
training is a kind of 'material thinking' (Carter 2004) in the body, which engages
action and reflection simultaneously. Whilst this might be true of any class, Tully's
method of teaching, developed outside established 'systems,' is distinct and refined.
He teaches dance as a classical art for all time, through movement principles that
are firmly rooted in physical laws relating to gravity and mass:

> a fundamental principle of the dance is the line of aplomb.[4] [...] This would
> be a principle *and* a natural law. The dancer by so establishing himself in

relation to the centre of gravity would have not only a centre, but a cir-
cumference also, a special dimension.

(Tully 2011:17, added emphasis)

His approach invites questions about the function *and* expression of the text or
form of the dance sequences that comprise the class structure. He theorizes the
centrality of the line of the aplomb thus,

> The line of aplomb implies a centre or still point from which movement
> may move out, to which it will return and which will be present through-
> out. 'En-dehors,' 'En-dedans,' 'En place': the outward movement, the in-
> ward movement, and being in place; these are the three great expressions
> of the classical dance.

(Tully 2011:17)

His precept that the 'geometries are acquired through experience' (Ibid.: 18) likewise invites mindful exploration of dancing according to principles, both how I
embody those principles and how they are embodied in the construction and form
of the sequences. Our practice stimulates discussion and learning goes on after class
over cups of tea. There is a tacit recognition that in the shared exploration and
flow between teacher and student, both personal and disciplinary knowledge and
understanding grows. In this artistic studio, the hierarchies of knowledge power
that are a function of ballet institutional systems of performance and training are
redundant and I saw the rich possibilities in the dialogue between my different
dance knowledges – as dancer, choreographer, teacher.

Studying in this environment with somatic (first-person) attention to the feeling of the geometry of the ballet forms has invited a deeper reflection about my
experience of the 'fundamental principles' in relationship to time.

Does attention to the aplomb teach about:

- the (expanded) time between the still point and movement;
- the place between balance and falling that I rehearse when standing in the
  aplomb and then moving outwards and inwards from the inferred centre;
- the moment that holds in potential the impulse to move, to step?

Does it teach that the beat of music only marks a step after the fall into gravity
from the aplomb; that my body must occupy its own architecture, and feel its *own*
time to be expressive of the dance itself?

Charles M. Joseph's biography of the great artistic collaboration between
Stravinsky and Balanchine cites physicist and cosmologist A. S. Eddington. 'We
often think that when we have completed our study of *one* we know all about
two because "two" is "one and one." We forget that we still have to make a study
of "*and*"' (2002:9; original emphasis). What might nurture the 'AND' between
training in ballet and creative development of choreographic forms that will

sustain its future life? Looking beyond class to the ballet stage, I observe that many talented dance-makers don't connect with ballet as a medium of *personal* expression. Class is a very personal practice, but the training can feel regimented and oriented towards athletic and technical outcomes. Technical development can be a satisfying aspect of engaging in the ballet class 'as body conditioning,' but may not lead to a deeper structural understanding of how the gestures are expressive in themselves and of an individual relationship with the ballet text.

When teaching choreography at the Royal Ballet School,[5] attention to stillness was an essential principle in our exploration of the 'Body as expressive instrument.'[6] Workshops followed a similar pattern – introduction of theme and ice-breaker, experiential guided improvisation, setting choreographic task, creating in response to the task, sharing and discussion. We would begin each experiential guided improvisation and sharing of material with stillness and in silence.

It places us in time:

> Everyone waits until the room is still. Many dancers find the simple still-ness exposing. It makes some dancers anxious. Being held in stillness is a clear contrast to the habit of consistently moving to the beat – which can become engrained in ballet class. The dancer has time to sense not only her own repose and alertness, but that of the others in the room. In the discipline of the moment she becomes aware of the rhythm of the space and being centred – the impulse for movement in her own body. She enters into an expanded relationship with the musical pulse or 'beat' and rhythm. Connected to her natural body along the line of the aplomb, poised in relation with gravity, time expands, she feels the moment, she feels time.[7]
>
> *(Jackson 14th October 2013)*

Alongside these observations of the choreography class, I have experienced a reawakening of the inner 'music' of my own dance, when participating in Tully's ballet class. The sequences of dance action seem to be initiated neither by movement or music, but arise simultaneously from the same 'place' of stillness. My response to dancing the material has changed: I am obedient to the given form and timing, but I sense the inner dynamic life of the movement and an expansion of time to play with accent and phrasing. I connect this inner dynamic to the way I experience the aplomb – giving time to sensing the weight or mass of my body (balance) and the reach of the limbs (kinesphere) in relation to my own physical centre. Paying close attention to my body weight and the subtle feeling of lightness along the line of the aplomb – the sense of 'poise' that is character-istic of a ballet dancer – I am both rooted and suspended along the vertical line of my skeletal (and architectural) structure. I experience stillness, a clarity and emptying of self that gives rise to awareness of movement from a deeper place.

In my experience, educating the dancer in the principle of aplomb resonates clearly with the pre-eminent choreographer Balanchine's ideas about time and expression in dance, and is pivotal. 'Music is something that occupies *architecturally* a certain portion of time. In the dance, unless your body fills time, occupies time, as music does, then it means nothing. Gesture is meaningless' (quoted in Joseph 2002: 8; added emphasis).

Class is the action research at the heart of the dancer's personal praxis. Canvassing fellow mature dancers, they *all* cite 'joy' as one reason for attending. One dancer strongly evokes the personal: 'It reminds me of who I am,' another 'the music of the body.'[8] My studies at university prepared me intellectually for embracing apparent paradoxes in ballet: a dance that is 'natural' *and* 'geometric.' My practice as a mature dancer is the joyful embodiment of paradox. I enjoy exploring beyond the naming of steps – ballet's 'five positions of the feet' are misconceived – the feet are merely indicators of the transfer of body weight. I am excited by the impossibilities of dancing 'in the body'[9] not 'on my legs.' Emotionally, Tully's studio has offered an environment for personal vulnerability and artistic growth, a space where process, questions and exploration of the forms speak back to the body, where at whatever age, I have the ideal body for my own dance. Because in my body, I enjoy sensing the aplomb, the stillness, the geometries, movement outwards and inwards – the feeling of occupying time, as music does.

Notes

1 Patrick Wood is an independent ballet teacher and choreographer. He began his dance training with Rambert School aged 20; danced with Festival Ballet, Scottish Ballet and in the West End and studied with Tully privately when learning to teach.

2 Regular attendees of Tully's class meet once a week in London. Tully (born 1928) continues to teach fortnightly and one of the dancers elects to teach from their personal understanding of the shared practice when Tully is not teaching.

3 My 2005 article 'My dance and the ideal body' is a detailed discussion of training the 'ideal body' in relation to the balletic concepts of *en dehors* and *en dedans*.

4 The concept of aplomb refers to the fundamental relationship of the dancer's physical centre with gravity and whilst also inferring an attitude of mind.

5 From 1999 to 2016, I worked with Kate Flatt, developing a course for teaching choreography at the Royal Ballet School, London. Flatt's background is as an educator and she is internationally known as a choreographer/director in theatre and opera. As a trainee teacher, she studied with ballet choreographer Leonide Massine and with Nina Fonaroff, renowned as Choreography Teacher at The Place.

6 In devising tasks for creating with the ballet form in choreography class, I elaborated on the states of being and associations sparked by the experience of 'inhabiting' the geometries of forms with somatic attention. Parallels between Tully's description of key balletic concepts, *en dehors*, *en dedans* and *en place*, with the way I was theorizing my choreographic understanding and practice are striking and are articulated in my 2008 paper: Jackson, J (2008) 'En place – choreographic investigations of the dancer's awareness of ballet form,' in C. Stock (ed.), *Dance Dialogues: Conversations across cultures, artforms and practices*, Proceedings of the 2008 World Dance Alliance Global Summit. Online publication, QUT Creative Industries and Ausdance, http://www.ausdance.org.au

7 For discussion of beat and pulse in relation to embodiment of rhythm in dancing, see Kaminsky, D. (2014) 'Total rhythm in three dimensions: Towards a motional theory of melodic dance rhythm in Swedish Polska Music,' *Dance Research* 32(1): 43–64.

8 Fellow dancers offered these comments after ballet class, 2 January 2018.

9 This is one of several of Tully's in class 'sayings' that describe experience in a way that resonates strongly.

References

Carter, P. (2004) *Material Thinking; The Theory and Practice of Creative Research*, Melbourne: Melbourne University Press.

Jackson, J. (2005) 'My dance and my ideal body,' *Research in Dance Education*, 6(1.2): 25–40.

——— (2008) 'En place – choreographic investigations of the dancer's awareness of ballet form,' in C. Stock (ed.), *Dance Dialogues: Conversations across cultures, artforms and practices*. Proceedings of the 2008 World Dance Alliance Global Summit. Online publication, QUT Creative Industries and Ausdance, http://www.ausdance.org.au

——— (2013) Choreography class observation notes, 14th October, Royal Ballet School, Upper School, Covent Garden, London. 2013.

Joseph, C.E. (2002) *Stravinsky and Balanchine; A Journey of Invention*, New Haven, CT and London: Yale University Press.

Kaminsky, D. (2014) 'Total rhythm in three dimensions: towards a motional theory of melodic dance rhythm in Swedish Polska Music,' *Dance Research*, 32(1): 43–64.

Tully, R. (2011) *The Song Sings the Bird: A Manual on the Teaching of Classical Dance*, Rome: Gremese.

14

THE DANCE OF OPPOSITION

Repetition, legacy and difference in Third Theatre training

Jane Turner and Patrick Campbell

Introduction

The term Third Theatre was coined in a short text written 40 years ago by renowned theatre director Eugenio Barba, founder of Odin Teatret – a pioneering theatre company established in 1964 and based in Holstebro, Denmark.[1] Barba used the term to describe an emerging generation of theatre groups in the 1970s who associated themselves neither with mainstream (First Theatre) nor avant-guard theatre (Second Theatre). According to Barba, marginality, autodidactism, the existential and ethical dimension of the craft and a new social vocation were the fundamental characteristics of this community.

From the 1970s to the present day, Third Theatre has refined itself as a multifarious, transnational entity, comprised of groups and solo artists across the world (but primarily in Europe and Latin America) making theatre in a laboratory environment in which training is generally an essential aspect of the practice. Many of these artists are border-crossers, working with colleagues from an array of different countries and backgrounds, often gathering periodically in order to reaffirm a collective identity and replenish themselves artistically. As this chapter will demonstrate, the Third Theatre community continue to celebrate and offer a 'time' and 'place' – a way of being together – to diverse, foreign[2] and unruly theatre practices. The ties linking this Third Theatre community are profound; despite recurring economic and financial constraints in their home countries, these artists continue to make work that shares common values and principles. Thus, the territory carved out by Third Theatre is as much temporal as it is spatial, characterized by intense periodic encounters, a privileging of continuous psychophysical training and the adoption of diverse dramaturgical techniques that foreground the embodied presence of the actor in performance. As Barba suggests,

In theatre, time is created artificially. One possibility: to imagine time is neither outside me nor does it flow around me: I am time, it is me who flows. Then time is no longer an abstract dimension, but it is matter endowed with senses, directions, impulses and rhythms. Time becomes a living organism which may be moulded into actions felt as rhythmical units by the spectator.

(2010: 195)

For the purpose of this chapter, we have chosen to focus on how time shapes and is manifest within the training processes of three artists who exemplify different aspects of the Third Theatre community: Luis Alonso,[3] Carolina Pizarro[4] and Mia Theil Have.[5] All three artists have continuing relations with Odin Teatret's sister organization Nordisk Teaterlaboratorium (NTL), which, amongst other responsibilities, nurtures and incubates young artists from the Third Theatre community. All three artists work on the margins of a varying array of geopolitical contexts, developing, through their work, what Levitt and Schiller have referred to as 'ways of belonging,' practices that '[…] signal or enact an identity which demonstrates a conscious connection to a particular group. These actions are not symbolic but concrete, visible actions that mark belonging' (2004: 1010). Belonging in the case of these artists refers to an affiliation with the wider Third Theatre community, its practices and ethos.

In many ways, their experiences reflect a new generation of Third Theatre artists, working in a globalized, mediated world, building on a small *interstitial* tradition in a mindful, respectful yet innovative way. By interstitial, we refer to a culture of practice that seeks to resist binaries and any notion of cultural purity. The interstitial exists in a *third space*, a locus where, according to Bhabha, '[…] the meaning and symbols of culture have no primordial unity or fixity; that even the same signs can be appropriated, translated, rehistoricized, and read anew' (Bhabha 1994: 21). Thus, the interstitial speaks to a number of different ways of being in-between (genres, cultures, groups) without privileging any one, and also acknowledges the sharing of points of contact. In this sense, an interstitial theatrical tradition is one of constant creative negotiation, acknowledging whilst challenging difference.

Our aim here is to investigate the temporal intricacies surrounding the interstitial training processes at the heart of these artists' practices. We shall do this by drawing on the artists' voices, whilst critically exploring how they articulate the importance and value of training in their daily practice. We are particularly interested in the complex play of embodiment, affective intensity and temporal lines of flight that colour the work of the actor as s/he develops his/her *craft*, understood as an autonomous, eclectic and continuing process of work on the self in relation to the theatrical event.

Deleuze's three syntheses of time

In terms of a critical framework for conceptualizing time, Deleuze's work around the three syntheses of time – *the living present*, *the pure past* and *the drive to the future* – developed primarily in his 1968 publication *Difference and Repetition* (reprinted in 1994), is of value for mapping out this complex territory from a philosophical perspective. Deleuze's philosophy of time focuses primarily on repetition and difference. The 1968 work is a critique of structuralist approaches to representation that operate at a level of fixity. By focusing on the essential difference underpinning all repetition, Deleuze is able to map out a process of constant 'becomings,' rather than fixed 'being' (see Deleuze 1994: 41). Importantly, there is a resonance here between this constant becoming, and the processual nature of performer training. How this functions in the particular case of the Third Theatre will become apparent in the next section. This ontology of becoming has important ramifications for the conceptualization of time. Deleuze's detailed examination of repetition and difference allows him to deconstruct causal models of temporal succession, and to propose three *syntheses* of time, broadly based on (a) habit, (b) memory and (c) the 'new', in which linear notions of past, present and future overlap and fold into one another. This temporal multiplicity importantly contradicts notions of the unity of time and of its unique direction from past to future.

In the first synthesis, 'the living present,' the past lingers and the future is an anticipated dimension of the present. This is the basic passive synthesis of time, which precedes memory and reflection (Deleuze 1994: 78). In terms of performer training, every time a performer steps into the space s/he is drawing on a practice and working this out in the present. This is the realm of habit; repetition opens up a living present for us. In the second synthesis, the 'pure past,' it is the flux of differences or becomings that are underpinning any possible embodied memory which are shown to be working incessantly on the present, engulfing it constantly (Deleuze 1994: 94). In other words, when working on a given exercise, embodied memory is an active force that can contaminate the present, and thus the present moment can be submerged within a pre-existent and coexistent flow of prior experiences of the Other – the lineage of artists whose bodies have already shaped this practice. Finally, in the third synthesis, the future is a novel event, the result of a defining 'cut' or caesura made possible by the ongoing 'eternal return' of pure difference in the present: the potential for differing assemblages of repeated processes to emerge (Deleuze 1994: 89). In training, this is the 'eureka' moment, where time is thrown out of joint; the artist breaks with the past, and renews tradition through the discovery of a novel form of exercise. Novelty here can be the repetition of the same exercise, but with a fundamental difference, a shift in intention and approach.

Time is thus manifest through multiple synthetic processes. However, Deleuze asserts that these syntheses are nevertheless *asymmetrical*; this means that rather than some form of atemporal soup, the progress of time is irrevocable. Whilst common sense notions of past, present and future constantly combine and fuse together in novel ways through differing syntheses of complex processes, the difference underpinning repetition makes for constant, irreversible change (Deleuze 1994). Whilst the particularities of this tripartite model will become apparent through our analysis of the artists' encounters with performer training, what is highly useful in Deleuze's conceptual account is the way in which it acknowledges the multiplicity of time and the fragmented nature of subjectivities, which are always shifting in relation to a passive 'larval' self – an unconscious self, immersed in different, highly complex and unruly processes. Time is the result of the syntheses of multifarious processes, and not the other way around. Importantly then, whilst one synthesis of time may be more dominant in the way in which a given artist may speak of his/her training, their embodied experiences reflect a complex interstitial weaving of all three temporal states.

Repetition is a key aspect of the continuous, prolonged approach to training in the Third Theatre tradition. However, in accord with Deleuze's thinking, whilst the repetition of daily training is necessarily habitual, it is also an active process of seeking *difference*. It is all too easy for the performer's body to become complacent and mechanistic, especially after years of working on the same principles day in, day out; the challenge is to constantly make new connections in the living present and rediscover the value of the training (as pure past) in the here and now, maintaining a vital, living process of discovery in which the future eruption of the novel is always a potentiality.

Repetition and difference – Luis Alonso and his involvement with the Bridge of Winds

Initiated by Odin actress Iben Nagel Rasmussen[6] in 1989, the Bridge of Winds is a closed group of about 20 performers from around the world who had all previously been participants in workshops led by Rasmussen. Luis Alonso is one of the members of this group, and joined the Bridge of Winds in 2005. He set up Oco Teatro Laboratório in Brazil alongside fellow Bridge of Winds member, Rafael Magalhães in 2003. In an interview with the authors, Alonso spoke particularly about the training undertaken with the Bridge of Winds and the continued importance this has for him in terms of his professional and personal development. The Bridge of Winds has been meeting annually for a 4-week period over the past 25 years. Each meeting sees the group working on set exercises on a daily basis for several hours without pause. The exercises are physically and mentally challenging: physically because they are arduous and mentally because they are repetitious and challenge the performer to constantly remain alert and connected (Figure 14.1).

La Selva, in her appraisal of the Bridge of Winds' training, states that it is evident that the form of the exercises and engagement with them by the group has been refined and could only have been devised through a '(very) long-term experience' (La Selva and Turosik 2015). La Selva describes the five key exercises that comprise the annual training regime[7]; here we are interested in examining one in particular: the 'Wind Dance.' As described by La Selva, the 'Wind Dance'

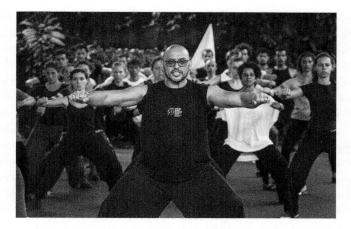

FIGURE 14.1   Luis Alonso working with the Bridge of Winds. Photo: Francesco Galli. Courtesy of Odin Teatret Archives.

[…] is a very simple step, present in many different cultures, based on the count of 3, like the waltz. Jump, right foot lands smoothly on the ground, toes first. No sound. Left foot joins the right one closely and for a moment, it pulls the body towards a vertical impulse. Right foot first, then left one lands, already pointing the next direction of the body. Exhaling, knees bend deeper, grounding our energy, receiving the power to restart.

(Idem.)

La Selva notes that this deceptively simple exercise does not have a rigid temporal and spatial structure, despite the fact that its outer form is fixed. She reports that Rasmussen emphasizes that for members of the group, it is important to deconstruct the exercises once they are back in their home countries and daily artistic routines, '[…] so when they meet again, they have the chance to rediscover, to re-territorialize the sources of their own poetics and practices' (Idem.). La Selva's observations, and particularly her emphasis on the reterritorialization of training exercises resonate with Alonso's account of his ongoing embodied dialogue with the Bridge of Winds. He describes his initial period of training with the group as being '[…] extremely hard; your body aches' (Alonso 2016). He defines it is as a moment of transgression because, '[…] as a performer, you are required to let go of your body and its training and let someone else in' (Idem).

A link can usefully be made here to the Deleuzian notion of the present as a dimension of the pure past: the actor, faced with the living memory, the full energetic intensity of an embodied training developed by seasoned practitioners over a period of years, encounters this initially as a physical shock before fully incorporating it as his own. Hastrup, writing about Third Theatre, describes this process as 'acculturation,' which is defined as '[…] the internalization of a new set of rules for action [...] the learning of a new presence' (Hastrup 1995: 78). Here, the passive, larval self is swept up in a wave of intensities ushered in by the processes underpinning the training. In order to make sense and incorporate this experience, the subjects find themselves in the living present, where the past is necessarily contracted, revisited and repeated. It is in this act of repetition that difference emerges, and the legacy is renewed and transformed.

Alonso speaks of the training today as a '[...] dance between the collective and the solitary; between prison and freedom' (2016). He sees this dialectic between apparent sameness and underlying difference as a necessary tension for the formation of the artist and the equilibrium of the group. What is significant to our argument here is that the notion of time and temporality experienced in this mode of repetition provides a sense of continuity. The fixed/knowable space of the 'Wind Dance' and the other exercises offers the members an opportunity to relocate a sense of their self, derived from a past experience that in each cycle of repetition is transformed; for core members of this group, they have been repeating the exercises for 25 years. Moreover, the necessity to somehow 'liberate' oneself whilst retaining the form entails a constant process of differentiation and creative subterfuge. The training is thus renewed whilst remaining constant.

Importantly then, the time and space defined by the annual meeting of the group can also be described, following Hastrup, as a 'social experience' (1995: 81); that is, an experience derived from the continuous and repetitious meeting of the members over a period of 25 years. Over this time, a unique transnational theatre community has been established that is set apart from other aspects of the members' professional lives and identities. Alonso describes the time, space and repetition of the training forms as a *liminal* experience, in which

> [...] you exist in an in-between space where you encounter the 'other' in yourself as well as performers other to yourself, who are from different cultures but importantly have all travelled and left their culture behind for the month of the training.
>
> *(Alonso 2016)*

Perhaps this sense of liminality is precisely a felt sense of the ways in which the training allows group members to work on a deeper level than the fragmented subjectivity Deleuze alludes to in *Difference and Repetition*. This fragmented subjectivity is cast in a binary embrace with the unconscious, passive larval self, which is constantly 'dissolving'; being worked upon by the processes defining time (Deleuze in Williams 2011: 93). This marks the transformational potential unlocked by the training; driven to extremes of tiredness and fatigue through physical rigour, coordination and energetic play, new embodied and affective connections are made, and the opportunity for decisive breaks, or encounters with novel expressive possibilities beyond the daily behaviour of the enculturated body is afforded. This caesura allows for the constant renewal of what may appear superficially as a fixed tradition of exercises.

It is the very mundanity and repetitious nature of these exercises that allow for creative discovery. Deleuze argues that this is because each repetition is always a variant and thus founded on a pure difference. Thus an act is always a variable of the past: '[…] just as fixed rules and a strategic pattern emerge, they lose their efficacy, forcing us to begin experimenting anew' (in Williams 2011: 91–92). For Alonso, as for the other members of the group, the Bridge of Winds offers a privileged time and space for the eternal return of difference in repetition, and thus harbours constant potential for artistic renewal and discovery.

Between the living present and the pure past – Carolina Pizarro's journey

Chilean-born Carolina Pizarro is an actress, director and teacher. After studying Theatre at university, she went on to develop an intense relationship with Odin Teatret, and in particular Odin actresses Julia Varley and Roberta Carreri, with whom she has trained and developed her solo practice. Challenged by Varley to develop her own training, she travelled to India, and spent a six-month period at the Hindustan Kalari Sangham Temple, where she developed her knowledge of Kalaripayattu and Silambattam martial arts. Pizarro went on to develop her own training, fusing Kalaripayattu with the tenets of Theatre Anthropology. In 2015, Pizarro was invited to join Odin Teatret as a permanent member of the ensemble. Thus, she has gone from being an independent artist carving out an autonomous path on the fringes of the Third Theatre to becoming an actress in an internationally renowned group with a 50-year heritage (Figure 14.2).

In terms of the interstitial nature of her training – which draws on Latin American and Asian forms, as well as the psychophysical training of different

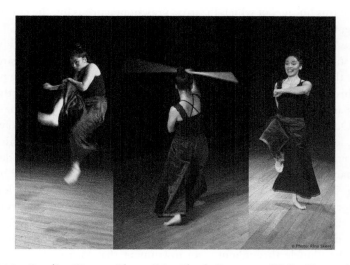

FIGURE 14.2 Carolina Pizarro. Photo: Rina Skeel. Courtesy of Odin Teatret Archives.

Odin actors, Pizarro states, '[...] whether I choose them or they choose me – I do not know ... They surprise me – and surprise me of my capabilities. I awaken things that I do not recognize in me' (2016). There is a resonance here between the surprise Pizarro feels at key moments in her training and the novelty of Deleuze's third synthesis – the rupture of the new as futurity. As in Alonso's case, the encounter with the fixed forms of codified movement practices can be liberating, as the artist discovers different energetic potentialities and trajectories through the body.

Whilst Alonso speaks of the training of the Bridge of Winds as a privileged liminal space, for Pizarro, her work as a solo artist and member of Odin Teatret has led to an experience and encounter with alterity as her interstitial practice opens up a play of sameness and deep difference; as subjective identity fades and she opens herself up to the affective potentiality of the training form, making constant holistic connections. She describes how, by moving away from her Latin American culture, she realized she was in her culture once again. To illustrate the point, she explains that she spent time with the Mapuche people in Chile, learning their dances. She recognized a similar consciousness to Kalaripayattu: both the Chilean dance and the Indian practice are connected to the earth, to nature and have a consciousness of fire. She says that 'without calling the Mapuche dance a meditation, it was like meditation' (Idem.).

Thus whilst Pizarro recognizes and respects cultural differences, there is also an embodied affective experience in the training that allows for connections to be made on a deep somatic level. From a Deleuzian perspective, perhaps there is a privileging here of the passive larval self, which allows itself to be worked upon by the flows of intensity that characterize the training. Thus, far from a simple cultural appropriation, Pizarro surrenders to these embodied practices as pure past, understood here as the continuing summation of all of the bodies that have passed on this lineage, of which Pizarro's present practice is but the current tip of the cone, to use Deleuze's visual metaphor of this temporal synthesis.

At the Third Theatre Network symposium developed by the authors in 2015,[8] Pizarro stated that 'the work is the master,' in response to questions regarding the status of the master in European theatre traditions. There is something powerful about this assertion; a recognition of the immaterial principals underlying the training as the ultimate guide for the self-reflexive actor. Moreover, having just joined Odin, Pizarro explains that her most recent training has involved very quickly, learning the performance scores of the group's repertoire. This has entailed having to create new material, whilst inserting herself into pre-developed performances by watching them on a DVD in the White Space, a working room at Odin. The material that Pizarro has had to learn for *Inside the Skeleton of the Whale* for example, incorporates the work of the previous three actresses who had developed the material for this role. In *The Chronic Life*, another Odin production, not only does she perform the whole piece blindfolded, but she also has to play the ukulele throughout – an instrument that Pizarro had no previous experience of (Idem.).

There is thus a tension present here between the privilege of joining Odin as a way of belonging, and the danger of being swallowed up by the deadliness of the past as a fixed entity. As in any lived tradition that a young performer immerses herself in, the past inevitably pervades the present of the practice; a legacy of intensities, of principals that are in fact transpersonal (and, in the case of Odin, cannot be reduced to the figure of the artist who perhaps initially founded the tradition). This is perhaps the challenge of any apprenticeship in any group; how to negotiate this loaded space between pure past and the living present.

Pizarro seems to achieve this through her continual energy, playfulness and openness. She synthesizes experiences constantly, encapsulated in this description of her personal training, which she undertakes whenever she gets the opportunity to return to her own practice beyond the context of performance preparation.

> More than exercises I work with principles – sequences of jumps with music, tiring the body and mind and then opening up – breaking the limits of 'I can't' and saying 'I can.' Spinning is very present; I think of Sufi dervishes and childhood – the earth spinning on its axis. Experiencing the body spinning and then the earth moving when you fall to the ground. There is a connection to the universe and to God. I want to recapture the energy and innocence of the play of childhood.
>
> *(Idem.)*

This spinning seems redolent of the living present, of this constant recycling of exercises and training and the potential chaos and disorder underpinning repetition. Pizarro's recreation of a childlike space evokes a sense of revitalization in the wake of tradition. Thus as an apprentice with Odin, she is located at the axial point of this process of renewal of an embodied tradition in the living present.

The cut – Mia Theil Have and riotous company

After working as a 'laboratory assistant' at Odin, Mia Theil Have participated as an actress in Theatrum Mundi performance *Ur-Hamlet*, linked to ISTA (the International School of Theatre Anthropology) and went on to join the Odin as a permanent member of the ensemble from 2004 to 2006, performing in *Andersen's Dream*, *The Great Cities Under the Moon* and *Don Giovanni all'Inferno*. After leaving the group, Have went on to carve out a career in London and internationally as a freelance director working in theatre and opera and founded her own company, Riotous Company, which now works in collaboration with Nordisk Teaterlaboratorium. Whilst Have says that she stands humble in front of established performance traditions, she also maintains a strong sense of self. Speaking of her time in Odin, whilst she constantly emphasized the richness of this experience, she states that, 'I always resist being subsumed. It is comfortable to be subsumed but let's not forget that I left the group. I left the group but evidently still need the relationship' (personal communication, March, 2016).

Have's path perhaps represents that which Deleuze describes as the 'cut,' or the caesura. She mentions that after leaving Odin, she discovered that she had a serious injury, which she struggled with for a number of years. Whilst this was a challenge, it also led her towards the freedom and independence she craved, enabling her to revisit the practice and the training on her own terms. Deleuze suggests:

> [...] the caesura, of whatever kind, must be determined in the image of a unique and tremendous event, an act which is adequate to time as a whole [...] Such a symbol adequate to the totality of time may be expressed in many ways: to throw time out of jolt, to make the sun explode, to throw oneself into the volcano, to kill God or the father. This symbolic image constitutes the totality of time to the extent that it draws together the caesura, the before and the after.
>
> *(Deleuze 1994: 89)*

This injury for Have was both shattering and liberating. The 'cut' here was literally embodied; Have had to accept the reality of her injured body rather than the virtuoso expectations placed upon the professional actress of physical theatre. This moment of crisis was her caesura and, for her, threw time 'out of jolt.' She began to engage with healing the body and returning to one of the roots of Third Theatre practice through its link to the Grotowskian tradition: yoga.[9] Have trained in Ashtanga Yoga during this period as a means of curing her injury, and went on to become a professional yoga instructor. She has made this practice an integral part of her performer training. According to Have, 'Ashtanga Yoga has allowed me to go deeper and [...] enabled me to work with my body in a holistic manner. Importantly, yoga is not about exterior expression – it is sustainable and is something I can trust' (personal communication, March, 2016).

As her injury has healed, Have has returned time and again to the training exercises she mastered whilst a pupil of Tage Larsen's and Else Marie Laukvik of Odin. She mentions the importance of Laukvik's compositional work to her practice, and also the stick work developed by Larsen in the 1970s. This latter training has importantly taken on an aesthetic dimension, and is at the core of Have's production for Riotous Theatre, *Scherzo for Stick* (2016), which is performed by Have and directed by Larsen. Thus, Have has carved out her own nomadic path. With a stick under one arm, and a yoga mat under the other, she has redefined the training she mastered at Odin, and has harnessed its nascent intentionality. Whilst she returns to her roots, this is always within the context of a process of transformation, revisiting the source of her training and simultaneously demarcating new territory.

Conclusion

Alonso, Pizarro and Have's practices are all characterized in different ways by refusal and the search for a personal meaning, which Barba suggests is the foundation of all Third Theatre (Barba 1991). According to Barba,

There exists an invisible revolt, apparently painless yet infusing every hour of work, and this is what nourishes "technique." Artistic discipline is a way of refusal. Technique in theatre and the attitude that it presupposes is a continual exercise in revolt, above all against oneself, against one's own ideas, one's own resolutions and plans, against the comforting assurance of one's own intelligence, knowledge, and sensibility.

(Barba 2000, 56)

Revolt is thus akin to the difference underpinning repetition in Deleuze. Whilst all of the artists are constantly enmeshed within Deleuze's three syntheses of time – these differentiated contractions and extensions of past, present and future – discursively, their testimonies allow us to tease out different temporal inflections in each of their journeys. Whether we focus on Alonso's sense of a liminal space beyond encultured subjectivity in the Bridge of Wind's training, Pizarro's surrender to the intensity of the Odin training as pure past and playful renewal of tradition in the living present or Have's decisive caesura and forward-moving intentionality with Riotous Company, all three artists mark out new paths for the future.

What this highlights is that the interstitial nature of Third Theatre allows for and accommodates difference, legacy and revolt. This space on the margins has a different tempo-rhythm to First or Second theatre, and is neither swayed by the product-orientated demands of commercial theatre, with its tight rehearsal periods or the fleeting fashions of the avant-garde. Importantly, Third Theatre allows for a way of belonging to an artisanal theatrical community with a strong ethos predicated on nurturing difference, allowing people to learn and unlearn and learn anew. There is space in Third Theatre to flow in and out of different temporal syntheses according to their own personal needs. The difficulty is maintaining this marginalized third space, which is far from utopian; there are constant material struggles to be negotiated, and all three artists have demonstrably had to dance to other tunes, finding a way to maintain their own sense of time and rhythm, whilst accommodating the demands of earning a living and establishing themselves in the arts. The ongoing future of Third Theatre depends on this balancing act.

Notes

1 For literature available on the praxis and history of Odin Teatret, see Barba (1999), Varley (2010), Carreri (2014), Watson (1995), Ledger (2012), Chemi (2018) and Turner (2018).

2 In Barba's writing, he uses foreign as a term to indicate a locus of professional practice and a necessity to remain at the margins of culture and traditions (see Barba 1986: 10).

3 https://www.thirdtheatrenetwork.com/?page_id=247.

4 http://www.odinteatret.dk/about-us/actors/carolina-pizarro.aspx.

5 https://www.riotouscompany.co.uk/company.

6 We acknowledge throughout this article the important role played by the actors of Odin Teatret in maintaining alive and supporting a tradition of culture amongst

the wider Third Theatre. From the 1970s, when Rasmussen and Larsen first began to adopt young pupils, all of the Odin actors have gone on to develop lasting pedagogical practices. However, a more in-depth discussion of these varied processes of knowledge transfer is beyond the scope of this present chapter.

7 Other exercises include 'Green' which is based on working with resistance; slow motion; 'out-of-balance' which maps onto Barba's pre-expressive elements of opposition and luxury balance; and finally 'samurai', which works with 'animus' energy, another pre-expressive element.

8 *A Handful of Dust: the praxis and diasporic legacy of Odin Teatret*. A Third Theatre Network event organized by the authors in collaboration with Manchester Metropolitan University and Odin Teatret/Nordisk Teaterlaboratorium, which took place at Contact Theatre Manchester from the 30–31st October, 2015.

9 Like Stanislavski before him, Grotowski also incorporated elements of yoga into the psychophysical performer training – see Schechner and Wolford (2001) *The Grotowski Sourcebook*. London: Routledge.

References

Alonso, L. (2016) Skype interview with authors.

Barba, E. (1986) *Beyond the Floating Islands*, New York: PAJ.

———— (1991) 'The Third Theatre. A legacy from us to ourselves', *New Theatre Quarterly*, 8(29): 3–9.

———— (1999) *Theatre: Solitude, Craft, Revolt*, Aberystwyth: Black Mountain Press.

———— (2000) 'A deep order called turbulence,' *The Drama Review*, 44(4) (T168): 56–66.

———— (2010) *On Directing and Dramaturgy*, London: Routledge.

Bhabha, H. (1994) *The Location of Culture*, London: Routledge.

Carreri, R. (2014) *On training and performance: traces of an Odin Teatret actress*, Abingdon: Routledge.

Chemi, T. (2018) *A Theatre Laboratory Approach to Pedagogy and Creativity. Odin Teatret and Group Learning*, Basingstoke: Palgrave Macmillan.

Deleuze, G. (1994) *Difference and Repetition*, Columbia: Columbia University Press.

Hastrup, K. (1995) *A Passage to Anthropology*, London: Routledge.

Have, M.T. (2016) Skype interview with authors.

La Selva, A. and Turosik, M. (2015) '25 years again and again: on time and articulated knowledge at The Bridge of Winds' group,'in Paper presented at Theatre and Performance Research Association (TaPRA), UK: University of Worcester.

Ledger, A. (2012) *Odin Teatret: Theatre in a New Century*, Basingstoke: Palgrave Macmillan.

Levitt, P. and Schiller, N.G. (2004) 'Conceptualising simultaneity: a transnational social field perspective on society,' *International Migration Review*, 38(145): 595–629.

Pizarro, C. (2016) Skype interview with authors.

Schechner, R. and Wolford, L. (2001) *The Grotowski Sourcebook*. London: Routledge.

Turner, J. (2018) *Eugenio Barba*, (2nd ed.), Abingdon: Routledge.

Varley, J. (2010) *Notes from an Odin Actress*, Abingdon: Routledge.

Watson, I. (1995) *Towards a Third Theatre*, London: Routledge.

Williams, J. (2011) *Gilles Deleuze's Philosophy of Time: A Critical Introduction and Guide*, Edinburgh: Edinburgh University Press.

SECTION V

Out of time

Beyond presence and the present

Out of time

Beyond presence and the present

15

BRIDGING MONUMENTS

On repetition, time and articulated knowledge at The Bridge of Winds group

Adriana La Selva

It is a very simple step, present in different cultures, based on the count of three, like the waltz. (1): Jump, right foot landing smoothly on the ground, exhaling. Toes first, no sound. (2): The left foot joins the right closely and, for a moment, pulls towards a vertical impulse, bringing the body to a small, fast spring, while inhaling. (3): Exhaling, the left foot lands, the knees bend deeper, grounding our energy to power a restart.

I invite the reader to take this step as a microcosm.

Developed over almost 30 years by Odin Teatret's actress Iben Nagel Rasmussen (1945–) and the members of The Bridge of Winds group, this step, called 'the wind dance,' contains, within a count of three, the whole of a relation to theatre, with the work of the actor and her ethos. With the whole of *a theatre*.

I joined The Bridge of Winds as an observer in their annual meeting in 2015 in Holstebro, Denmark. Through my engagement with the meetings that followed, I slowly began to take part in all their activities (training, performances, production, research), working closely with Rasmussen and other group members. This chapter draws on this experiential perspective, further supported by a series of interviews with members of the group. As the lifelong work of The Bridge of Winds members focuses on cultivating the actor's qualities – a cultivation experienced as a continuous and resistant action – presence is here understood as an ethical process unfolding through repetition. The key aim of the chapter is precisely to investigate the relation between long-term repetition, creation and the performer's ethos. This relation is analysed through Gilles Deleuze's conceptualization of repetition and difference within his ontology. Framing the territory through Deleuze's writings highlights a specific view on repetition as a key principle of engaging in an alternative working model, one that articulates different deployments of time as a creative and resistant force in the actor's work, and challenges neoliberal paradigms of performer training (Figure 15.1).

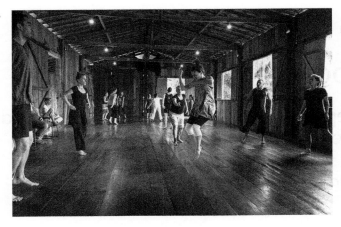

FIGURE 15.1 Exploration of the wind dance in two groups, 2016 © Francesco Galli.

Building up a bridge

The Bridge of Winds is an international theatre group, incorporated into the Nordisk Teaterlaboratorium in Denmark, which is also the home of Odin Teatret. The group was born out of Rasmussen's desire to transmit and explore her tacit legacy on actor training, in parallel with her work with Odin.

Rasmussen's artistic emancipation started when she felt the need to find her own path within the pre-expressive work that Odin Teatret was developing.[1] She was the first to join the group after their arrival in Holstebro (1966), where they have been based since then. After four years of committed dedication to the techniques that director Eugenio Barba was investigating with Odin, Rasmussen began to question their efficiency for her. She recounts how tired she would get from the practices and how hard it was to find the *continuous flow* that was so clear in other performers. In an interview with Barba (Rasmussen and Barba 2000), she speaks specifically of the work of actors Ryszard Cieślak (1937–1990) from Jerzy Grotowski's Teatr Laboratorium, and of Else Marie Laukvik (1944–) and Torgeir Wethal (1947–2010) from Odin; this *continuous flow* is what Rasmussen understands as the *transparent body*: a body that, through its physicality, becomes transparent, in order to 'let something else appear.' From this point on, Rasmussen began to ask what could work for her. What is, *for her*, a dramatic action. Through this questioning, she became convinced of the importance of transforming, adapting and recreating one's own training to reach autonomy over one's own creative work. This grew into a defining aspect of her relation to Barba's work since then. As Virginie Magnat observes,

> Not only is Rasmussen's perspective on the performer-director collaboration necessarily more fruitful from a creative standpoint, but it also means that when the performer becomes the owner of the modes of production,

so to speak, her labor of embodiment constitutes an investment in her own self, leading to an accumulation of cultural capital, or expertise, that sets her free from the wants, whims, and woes of her colleagues, critics, and public.

(2014: 105)

She then gathered a group of students she had met during previous workshops around the world and began to reconsider her pre-expressive work. Under her leadership, in 1989 they created a group of approximately 20 members that has been meeting every year for a session of two or three weeks, in a different location each year.[2] From the outset, her proposal was clear: to work with a fixed group of people on a long-term process, creating a dilated relation to/through time that allows a deep – though intermittent – development of their research.

The parts of the group's work that are perhaps most visible to the audience are their performances and barters.[3] However, from an insider's perspective, their most remarkable activity is the practice of a very specific voice and body training that facilitates and underscores their performative work. The group's discipline, their will to engage in the training every morning for the duration of the encounters, their driven repetition of a structure of exercises, overcoming the exhaustion that their (not-so-young-anymore) bodies endure, all constitute a training work at the limits of performativity.

The working structure is simple, respected and always agreed beforehand. The group has undoubtedly a master figure, Rasmussen, alongside many trainees who have been working long enough to assume the position of masters themselves. During the annual meetings, we meet daily and punctually to start the training. After some time warming up, a song sung together in a circle announces the beginning of the session. In the morning, we work without interruption on a devised sequence of exercises we all know by heart, accompanied either by the violin of musician Elena Borte Floris or by songs we sing together, songs from the different cultures of the group's members. The songs generate a dramaturgy for the progression of the training in time, giving us cues for moments of interaction, for changes in energy or in the space.[4] Rasmussen watches, takes notes and, at the end, provides brief comments regarding precision and energy. Nevertheless, when asked what she looks for in the training, she only replied: 'Connection' (La Selva and Rasmussen 2015). Afternoons are dedicated to the creation of new performances, concerts and barters throughout the region in which we set residence.

Watching the group first, and now working with them, crucial questions around time and temporality emerge. The members of the group live and operate within a neoliberal socio-political context, defined by market laws and the constant demand for immediate, short-term results, making this type of commitment to intermittent but recurrent training almost impossible to achieve. Yet, it seems that the group has found a 'gap' in this system, a 'way out,' prompting me to understand their work as a spatio-temporal site for resistance. What is the key for establishing this kind of long-term cooperation between such different artists, meeting for almost 30 years to practise work that is seemingly the same?

The simple rules (everything is in everything)

The group's tools have been distilled in five different kinds of exercises. Mika Juusela, one of the members, explains:

> These energetic exercises may have simple external form, but they are rather difficult to master. They are very precise and structured in a sequence that does not change much. It is a training that asks for a great amount of alertness, sensitivity and willingness to overcome one's physical comfort.
>
> *(La Selva and Juusela 2015)*

The group's work is sustained by the intriguing idea that one could find much of the tools needed to awaken the extra-daily body in very few exercises. And the will to master them so precisely has produced a certain training style that one could only create through a committed and repetitious long-term experience.

Each of these five exercises was devised to cultivate a specific working energy. The exercises evoke specific corporeal states from which the performers learn to draw their theatrical presence, the sources to create. The exercises are: (1) 'the wind dance' (the dance step described in the opening section, repeated for a long period and unfolding into many variations connected to simple daily actions); (2) 'green' (the practice of moving against a given resistance located in specific parts of the body, first experienced through stripes of cloth around the head, chest, heaps or knees, held by a partner moving behind the actor. Then, the actor is let free to move without the stripes, but holding the same movement quality provided by the resistance); (3) 'slow motion' (a rather complex way of moving, which, contrary to the 'green' exercise, works with no resistance. We aim for a continuous flow that Rasmussen sometimes describes as a 'seaweed dance'); (4) 'out of balance' (the body is brought out of balance and, just before it falls, moves to an opposite direction, so the energy that was supposed to end in a collision with the floor is thrown back into the space); and (5) 'samurai' (drawn from Japanese Noh techniques, it is the combination of, and variations on, three steps first learnt holding a stick with both hands in front of the body. These steps can be combined in 'fighting' interactions between the actors, including moments of attack, defense and retraction. The sticks are then taken away, providing more freedom for the arms. Nowadays, the samurai moves, which are related to a strong 'masculine,' open, yang energy, are integrated with '*gueixa*' energy: 'feminine,' closed, yin. While the samurai demands the whole body to engage in all the 'fighting' steps, the *gueixa* works with segmentation of specific body parts) (Figure 15.2).

Even though their outer forms are fixed, the exercises do not have a rigid temporal and spatial structure. This provides a great deal of freedom to investigate the relations we can build between us.

The group has been through a long path of learning through many other exercises before arriving at this training format. Although the exercises are fixed in terms of form, Rasmussen emphasizes an emancipatory process within the investigative environment: it is important that the members rethink and deconstruct these exercises once they are back in their home countries and artistic routines, so when we meet again, we have the chance to rediscover, to re-territorialize the sources of our own poetics and practices. In this sense, the apparent rigidity of this current structure becomes a place we can always come back to, a necessary home.

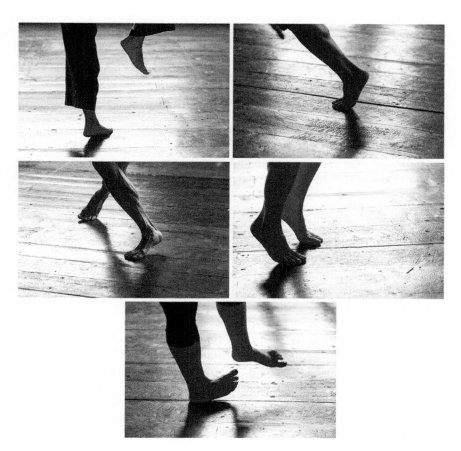

FIGURE 15.2   Feet close-up in the out-of-balance exercise, n01/02/03/04/05, 2016
© Francesco Galli.

Repetition, excess, becoming

Repetition features principally in the group's training ethos. Ethos, for Barba, is both 'a scenic behavior, that is, physical and mental technique' and a 'work ethic, that is, a mentality modeled by the environment and the human setting, where the apprenticeship develops' (2005: 278). The five exercises, repeated until body and mind reach a state of exhaustion, steer the group towards their creative processes, towards a theatre where forms, figures, characters, relations and encounters constantly actualize. What becomes enhanced, then, is presence. Not only as an extra-daily quality, but a presence that resonates throughout as an attitude towards daily life and the other. In this sense, there are two different but symbiotic ways of understanding the notion of presence, engaging with two notions of time, respectively: presence as an extra-daily quality – oriented towards performative purposes within specifically demarcated temporal frames and achieved through recurring periods of training – and presence as a daily, ongoing, temporally inexhaustible attitude, as an ethos.

Jori Snel, another member of the group, defines the forms they work with as 'the carriers' (La Selva and Snel 2015). The process of discovering what lies inside these forms is one that demands time and maturity. The process might even seem pointless at times as repetition does not succeed in exceeding itself without a great risk of getting bored or feeling empty along the way. Pulling oneself out of this risk demands sustained faith and patience. It has to become a sort of meditative practice on the 'cultivation of presence' (La Selva and Snel 2015).

Guillermo Angelelli, founding member of the group, describes the process of repetition as a 'sort of ritual and a work of faith' (La Selva et al. 2015). A faith on the techniques you have chosen to master, as they will lead you to the forms of expression, to the poetics you have been looking for, as long as the trainee faces and accepts the discipline of repetition: 'When you know a form, then you don't have to worry about this anymore and you can look further. This is for me the very importance of repeating' (La Selva et al., 2015).

Piotr Woycicki reminds us that scientists have found a neurological 'metronome' in the brainstem (2009: 80). This metronome is responsible for the stimulation of corporeal synchronic and automatic movements; simultaneously, it maps and inscribes these motion commands within our personal and cultural habits. When the body engages in continuous repetitive movements, this metronome is vulnerable to the generation of 'failures' within the commands executed, a process that is commonly the result of both physical and mental exhaustion. These 'failures' can be one of the most legitimate sources of creativity in theatre. In my practical experience with The Bridge of Winds, I have come to find within these 'failures' the most concrete bridge between pre-expressivity and expressivity, a place in between where technique meets creation. Woycicki defines these 'failures' as 'performance excess': 'an offset against the initial structure' (2009: 81), the unexpected – which is to say the very difference within repetition.

Gilles Deleuze's ontology of difference provides a rich theoretical foundation towards an anti-representational notion of movement in theatre. He envisions a theatre based on the 'power of becomings,' developed through operations of repetition.

> The theatre of repetition is opposed to the theatre of representation, just as movement is opposed to the concept and to representation which refers it back to the concept. In the theatre of repetition, we experience pure forces, dynamic lines in space which act without intermediary upon the spirit, and link it directly with nature and history, with a language which speaks before words, with gestures which develop before organised bodies, with masks before faces, with spectres and phantoms before characters – the whole apparatus of repetition as a 'terrible power.'
>
> *(Deleuze 1994: 10)*

Deleuze's theatre of repetition speaks of an operation that happens within the expressive moment itself, involving the *mise-en-scène* and the spectator's experience, 'the theatrical space, the emptiness of that space, and the manner it is filled and determined by the signs and masks' (1994: 10). However, when examined in the context of training, this operating machine he seeks *in expression* demands a perhaps even more powerful *pre-expressive* machine to allow this 'terrible power' to emerge from the apparatus of repetition. This 'terrible power' relies on the creation of difference within repetition, or 'performance excesses.'

Deleuze's non-systematic thinking is based on improvised concepts 'which are not always meant to be clear,' as if a concept should not be the definition of something, 'but a certain way of articulating complexities, as if to avoid closure or resolution' (Bruns 2007: 703). Further, he sees the individuation of an organism as determined by its potentialities, by its capacity to go through relations and transitions: 'we know nothing about a body until we know what it can do' (Deleuze and Guattari 1980: 284). Deleuze insists that his ontology is meant to be experienced in the body, something that has made his work an important reference for contemporary performing arts.

His writings cultivate a sustained interest in movement patterns and how they can be used to disrupt the organization of the body. Furthermore, Deleuze's ontology is that of process: organisms are considered in terms of their relationships to one another, their movement and their capacity to affect and be affected rather than as solo creatures, as stratified living beings. The actualization of an organism happens through a simultaneous and intrinsic set of complex relations, unreeled on what Deleuze calls *plane of immanence* (Deleuze and Guattari 1980: 281).

The *plane of immanence* works as a set of *latitudes* and *longitudes*, which are a determined set of *speeds* and *affects* that create specific energies. This configuration constitutes Deleuze's notion of a body: a body without organs, a body in potential. The (virtual) potentialities of the body, when actualized, are called *becomings*. As events, they do not sustain themselves; therefore, they do not stratify.

They happen by means of opening the body to relationships, creating *alliances* with other bodies. These *alliances* produce intensities called *affects*. *Becomings* are *affects in relation*. Our bodies, then, 'cease to be subjects to become events' (Deleuze and Guattari 1980: 262).

An important tool to actualize the body and produce becomings is the process of repetition. According to Slavoj Žižek, Deleuze's concept of repetition relies on the difference between mechanical and machinic repetition. While the first produces events of 'linear causality,' the latter (a 'proper' instance of repetition), instigates an event to be 're-created in a radical sense: it (re)emerges every time as New' (2004: 15).

In The Bridge of Winds, both in the practice and in terms of the ethos of the practice, the body becomes a plane of immanence, designed to facilitate encounters, affects, becomings through the apparatus of repetition. While engaging in the exercises through exhaustive repetition, I felt I could come very close to unknotting a place where several key notions Deleuze used to map his ontology meet. The plane of immanence, which is the body where becomings happen, is constituted of patterns of speeds and slowness, of patterns of energy.

Just as in many oriental physical traditions, The Bridge of Winds' exercises assume that some movements and positions can affect the overall organization of the body, transforming the notion of energy into objective matter, a palpable tool at hand to achieve a certain quality of presence. The rigorous training of the group not only puts the performer in touch with such patterns/energies, but also stimulates their manipulation and maintenance. Take the 'wind dance' as an example. As described in the introduction, the dance, based in a three-step movement, sets my body in a different organization: I have only one foot touching the ground, in relation with a precise way of breathing and dealing with my gravitational centres. To create the lightness of the wind in my movement, I need to be aware of the weight shifts during the jumps and the landings back on the ground. This constant change of weight and gravitational centres deterritorializes my body away from its ordinary balance, improving my awareness and sensibility. From this different awareness, I enter a relation with the group, and so the 'wind dance' becomes a tool to be manipulated in connection to the others and the space. Games begin to appear; *alliances* between bodies that can then affect the 'wind dance,' producing different speeds, actualizing – through repetition – the plane of immanence set by the exercise. The movement sustains the energy.

In the 'green exercise,' however, the energy sustains the movement. Energy is a set of inner tensions I need to constantly produce and renew to bring out a certain form and way of moving, based on a resistance against the space, as if this was filled with a thicker matter than air. This set of tensions, based on a gravitational centre rooted towards the ground, demands deeply bent knees and a way of walking so that my feet slide. This slows me down, restrains my outer forms, and is physically very demanding because of the amount of effort required to sustain the inner tensions created. Repetition appears here as a subtler element, a constant rearrangement of physical tensions demanding different kinds of concentration, with eyes turned to the inside. The exercise, consequently, becomes a more solitary experience, even in group work. Alliances have to be made first with myself, in an obsessive search for actualizing resistances.

Engaging with these exercises provokes a certain thinking attitude towards my craft: how can repetitive long-term practices of resistance, energy manipulation, alliances, becomings and affects frame an ethical attitude towards creation?

The macrocosm: a subtle provocation

This is a work that is quite exceptional, as the demands of theatrical production and related market laws do not provide the time necessary to construct a legacy of training research. Other European theatre groups that share a working philosophy similar to that of The Bridge of Winds, building long-term research on theatre practices and training, include, for instance, Gardzienice, Teatr ZAR, Teatr Pieśń Kozła (Poland), Attis (Greece), Farm in the Cave (Czech Republic) and Duende (UK).[5] These companies could be inserted in the context Barba named the Third Theatre:

> their theatre is neither what might be called avant-garde or experimental, not traditional, that is, part of a cultural institution. While their training has always been concerned with experimentation it is not experimental, in the sense that it is not concerned with challenging the boundaries of what might be considered acting. Its aim is to research, consolidate and refine the actor's craft. [...] The company sets itself very high standards for both their training and performance work, which are consistently rigorous and demand a discipline that is exacting.
>
> *(Turner 2004: 16)*

Such groups also share a different view on what being contemporary means. For Barba, much current theatre falls into a production formula that reflects what he calls *the spirit of the times*, 'an agenda imposed by a political regime or ideology' (Turner 2004: 8), consequently transformed into aesthetic tendencies, recurrent thematics and modes of creation pressed for time as economics become increasingly oppressive.

On the other hand, the idea of contemporaneity in relation to a group like The Bridge of Winds, which has been on the road for that long, demands an entirely different approach to what lives in the present and to what acts in the now, as their presence in the artistic landscape goes far beyond a repertoire of performances. Their exercises, already transmitted globally by second- and third-generation apprentices, constitute an ethical attitude to sharing *a* time together, engaging in exhaustive search for renewed connections and relations. This approach to training constructs an ethics and aesthetics of existence, turning practice into a way of participating in the present.[6]

In what sense, then, do these long-term training processes become sites of resistance to the ongoing imperative for novelty in contemporary performance, at times when ideas of innovation and creativity serve the production of a certain 'difference' demanded by the market itself to keep consumption going (Quilici 2015: 31)? Without dismissing the crucial importance of innovation in art production, I reference Žižek to propose that the *imperative* for novelty reproduces a mechanical repetition of forms, whereby the *representation* of difference appears as consumable goods imposed by 'the spirit of the times.' In contrast, the notion of repetition proposed here claims a radical view on newness, through structured practices acknowledged as research objects, prone to manipulation and transmission: 'it is not only that repetition is (one of the modes of) the emergence of the New – the New can only emerge through repetition' (Žižek 2004: 12).

Contemporary performance and, most importantly, contemporary *performers* have critiqued this repetitive aspect of training related to craft. Woycicki notes:

> The emphasis on craft honed through repetitiveness, together with the heavily institutionalized character of the way it is implemented and evaluated, have inspired much criticism from more 'intellectualized' approaches to methodology in arts practice. Such approaches often see this disciplining of the production of the sign through training as something limiting and anti-innovative – greatly compromising the agency of the performer/artist, merely recapitulating dominant conventions and standards in art.
>
> *(2009: 80)*

However, for The Bridge of Winds, training has become a way *out of* the disciplining of signs, providing each group member with significant freedom to search for their own theatrical poetics. Instead of leading to a compromise of my agency as a performer, experiencing these practices provided me with a specific ethical, political and performative discourse, which questions the regimes of creation criticized above, bringing me to think of practice as related to something greater than theatre itself, as something closer to the building of a monument that vibrates throughout time.

Monument, a concept introduced by Deleuze and Guattari to bridge the gap between their ontology and works of art that resonate with it, is an 'act by which the compound of created sensations is preserved in itself' (1994: 164). Monuments do not rely on materiality but in sensation and vibration, or rather, their materiality is built upon affects and becomings. As Deleuze and Guattari assert, a monument

> is not the commemoration, or the celebration, of something that has happened; instead, it confides to the ear of the future the persistent sensations embodying an event [...]. But the success of a revolution resides only in itself, precisely in the vibrations, embraces and openings it gives to men

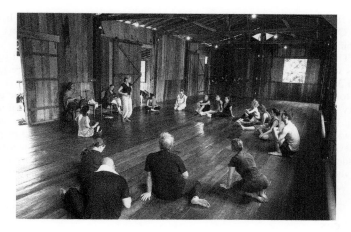

FIGURE 15.3 After training feedback, 2016 © Francesco Galli.

and women at the moment of its making and that composes in itself a monument in the constant process of becoming.

(1994: 176)

The coexistence between the various modes of repetition The Bridge of Winds
engage with (the wind dance step, the five exercises, the structured training sequence and the intermittent meetings throughout the past 30 years) gives form
to these affects and becomings, materializing such a monument, one that fosters
the resistant ethos promulgated by the group. This monument pushes me to
conceive of a practice moving beyond the (economic) structure of theatre itself.
It encompasses a way of understanding what the role of the performer in contemporary society is, a way of living together and expanding the borders of a shared
knowledge that dialogues with the passage of time.

One exercise, one action and the world in it (Figure 15.3).

Notes

1 Barba defines pre-expressive as 'The [performer's working] level which deals with
how to render the actor's energy scenically alive, that is, with how the actor can
become a presence which immediately attracts the spectator's attention' (Barba and
Savarese 2005: 188). For Rasmussen's training history within the Odin, refer to
Rasmussen (2018).
2 Rasmussen's pedagogical experience outside Odin began in 1983, with the creation
of the group Farfa. Before dissolving, the group also developed extensive training
research and many performances.
3 A theatrical barter is 'an event in which actions are the currency of exchange' (Watson
2002: 94), including demonstrations of particular skills (artistic, technical, sportive,
culinary, etc.) related to the participants' cultural background. This working format,
largely developed by Odin in the early 1990s, has allowed them to build a special
relation to communities beyond regular audiences, be it in a Syrian refugee camp,
an area of indigenous peoples on the Amazon or a remote rural area in Denmark.
The Bridge of Winds follows this tradition as part of their yearly meetings.

4 For a full account of the training structure and the exercises, visit http://livestream. com/OdinTeatretLiveStreaming/thebridgeofwinds. The video documents an open session during their 2015 meeting in Holstelbro.
5 The Third Theatre network stretches far beyond Europe, with significant representatives in other continents. This term resonates particularly with theatre groups in Latin America (see Watson 1987).
6 See, for example, the work by Carlos Simioni, a founding member of the group, in Paraty, Brazil with the Ateliê de Pesquisa do Ator – APA (Actor's Research Workshop). Under the leadership of Simioni and Stéphane Brodt (France), the workshop follows a similar model to that of The Bridge of Winds: a fixed group of performers develop a long-term research in training methodologies, during meeting blocks spread throughout the year. The Bridge of Winds exercises have now been appropriated and transformed according to their own cultural and political contexts. See also http://atelieator.blogspot.be/.

References

Barba, E. and Savarese, N. (2005) *A Dictionary of Theatre Anthropology: The Secret Art of the Performer*, New York and Oxon: Routledge.

Bruns, G.L. (2007) 'Becoming-Animal (some simple ways),' *New Literary History,* 38(1): 703–20.

Deleuze, G. (1994) *Repetition and Difference*, New York: Columbia University Press.

Deleuze, G. and Guattari F. (1980) *A Thousand Plateaus: Capitalism and Schizophrenia*, London: Continuum.

Deleuze, G. and Guattari F. (1994) *What Is Philosophy?* London: Verso.

Galli, F. (2016) *The Bridge of Winds: An Experience of Theatrical Pedagogy with Iben Nagel Rasmussen*, unpublished documentary.

La Selva, A. and Juusela M. (2015) 'Interview with Mika Juusela,' Holstebro, Denmark.

La Selva, A. and Rasmussen, I.N. (2015) 'Interview with Iben Nagel Rasmussen,' Holstebro, Denmark.

La Selva, A. and Snel, J. (2015) 'Interview with Jori Snel,' Holstebro, Denmark.

La Selva, A., Turosik, M. and Angelelli, G. (2015) 'Interview with Guillermo Angelelli,' Holstebro, Denmark.

Magnat, V. (2014) *Grotowski, Women and Contemporary Performance: Meetings with Remarkable Women*, New York: Routledge.

Rasmussen, I.N. (2018) *The Blind Horse: Dialogues with Eugenio Barba and Other Writings*, Ghent: Adriana La Selva.

Rasmussen, I. N. and Barba, E. (2000) 'The transparent body,' in Coloberti, C. (ed.), http://www.odinteatretarchives.com/thearchives/the-audiovisual-archives/examples/video-the-transparent-body1-2000.

Quilici, C.S. (2015) *O Ator-Performer e as Poéticas da Transformação de Si (The Actor-Performer and Self-Transformation Poetics)*, São Paulo: Annablume.

Turner, J. (2004) *Eugenio Barba*, Oxon: Routledge.

Watson, I. (1987) 'Third Theatre in Latin America,' *The Drama Review,* 31(4): 18–24.

——— (2002) 'The dynamics of barter,' in Watson, I. (ed.) *Negotiating Cultures: Eugenio Barba and the Intercultural Debate*, Manchester, MA: Manchester University Press, 94–111.

Woycicki, P. (2009) 'Repetition and the birth of language,' *Performance Research,* 14(2): 80–84.

Žižek, S. (2004) *Organs without Bodies: On Deleuze and Consequences*, London: Routledge.

16

THE ALWAYS-NOT-YET/ALWAYS-ALREADY OF VOICE PERCEPTION

Training towards vocal presence

Konstantinos Thomaidis

The here(-and-now?) of vocal presence: an onset

'In the uniqueness that makes itself heard as voice, there is an embodied exist-ent, or rather, a "being-there" [*esserci*] in its radical finitude, here and now': this affirmation launches the central chapter in Adriana Cavarero's philosophical treatise on voice (2005: 173; original emphasis). Out of this discursive onset, an argument is advanced in favour of a vocal ontology of uniqueness, a recognition, that is, of each singular being's sonorous materiality. Key to Cavarero's project is a disentanglement of voice from Derridean presence – as unavoidably different from itself and perpetually differed – through a committed attentiveness to vocal particularity. It is not surprising, then, that the epigraph by Walter Ong imme-diately preceding Cavarero's opening statement reads: 'Since sound indicates an activity that takes place "here and in this moment," speech as sound establishes a personal presence "here and in this moment"' (in Cavarero 2005: 173). While such consideration of embodied particularity – in other words, the 'being-*here*' of presence – is readily discernible as a quotidian preoccupation of voice peda-gogy for actors, the temporal constitution of vocal presence – its 'being-*now*' or 'being-*in-this-moment*' – might be less immediately circumscribed.

In performer training, presence is ubiquitously discussed in terms denot-ing 'here-ness,' terms primarily linked to a visual understanding of the body or space, with vocality an adjacent, if not occasionally subordinate, concern.[1] Among the rare works by practitioners that explicitly address voice as central to the issue of presence, Patsy Rodenburg's publications also embrace a visuocentric understanding of vocality in schematizing different levels of presence as operat-ing within three distinct circles of energy. As a First Circle speaker, for example, you are 'withdrawing physically' and you 'hide your visibility' (2007: 18), while, if habitually occupying the Third Circle, 'you take up more space than you need' (2007: 19). Presence is to be found in the Second Circle: you feel 'centered and alert' and that 'your body belongs to you,' while people 'hear you when you speak' (2007: 21).[2] With most voice pedagogues productively engaging the lexicon of visuality, with the 'now' of the 'here-and-now' of vocal presence routinely relegated to the 'here' or seemingly pronounced under one's breath, the temporal aspects of actors' vocal presence remain conspicuously unexamined.

As a first step towards tackling vocal presence *also* as a matter of time, the proposed strategy here is to attend to a particularly crucial moment in voice training: listening to one's own voice while in the act of voicing. The complexity of such a moment, for both trainees and educators, requires closer examination of the shaping of vocality during training, a process actively engendering and deeply affected by embodied understandings of time. In my attempt to listen-in to the makings of temporally present-ful voicing, the methodological point of departure is twofold. This chapter interweaves a phenomenological approach, which considers being-in/being-with as a temporal phenomenon related to presence, with a series of interviews conducted with six experienced teachers of voice in UK educational settings: Jane Boston, Deborah Garvey, Pamela Karantonis, Lisa Lapidge, Anna-Helena McLean and Daron Oram.[3] All interviewees primarily train actors; their backgrounds collectively represent various approaches to voice pedagogy, from 'natural voice' to classical singing and post-Grotowskian lineages of training.[4] Alongside conducting practice-led research, they are all actively involved in theatre practice as actors, singers, composers, music directors, voice coaches or performing poets. Our exchange explored definitions of vocal presence as emerging in the studio, the generation of exercises specifically designed to instil skills in presence, and the interconnections between control, presence and self-perception. This chapter draws on the interview extracts as generative entry points – rather than as exhaustive accounts of each respective practice.[5] My aim in entering into discussion with fellow voice practitioners was to examine the fundamental temporal presuppositions embedded in current voice training and ask: What can be revealed through researching the temporal attributes of trained vocal presence? What emerges through a re-temporalization of vocal presence? Which are the epistemic advantages of re-attuning vocal presence to its present?

When is the present of vocal presence? The time of voicing-listening/listening-voicing

When asked about definitions of vocal presence or whether they have developed a definition of vocal presence for the specific purposes of their studio work, all interviewees admit the complexity or impossibility of the task. 'In all honesty, I haven't defined the notion of vocal presence,' states Lapidge, and explains that she's more interested in discussing with students 'what it *could be*' (2018; original emphasis). If 'every definition of voice is a working definition' (Thomaidis 2015b: 214), divergence and incongruence are to be expected, and proposed solutions vary in correlation with vocal function, pedagogic setting and style/aesthetics. Impossible as vocal presence may seem to grasp, the trainers, rather than resisting or abolishing the term altogether, concur that it is a pervasive principle and overarching objective of their practice: 'at a macro level, the entire trajectory of training layers in' (Oram 2018) and 'all ones, vocal and singing exercises, are driving towards this aim' (McLean 2018). Lapidge also acknowledges: 'whilst I offer no firm definition, if someone were to ask me if I would want my actors to have "vocal presence," then I am convinced I would say "yes"' (2018). These potentially messy, sticky and contradictory ways of thinking about presence resonate with the micro-phenomenal experience of voicing, which – as will be argued throughout this section – embraces the present as a central aspiration of the training and, simultaneously, sets into motion a shift in emphasis towards its embodied future and past.

The complexities of embodiment are encapsulated in Boston's definition; she proposes a tripartite formula inclusive of 'physiological, psychological [factors] and acoustic variables' (2018). From a psychological point of view, the aim of voice pedagogy is tension release, freedom, liberation from blocks, alongside a 'preparedness to engage in the purpose of the vocal task' (Boston 2018). McLean also aims at a liberated voice without inhibitions and further points to the concrete aural qualities of such liberation: vocal presence is experienced as 'resonant sound that generates harmonics in the given acoustic' (2018). Garvey, too, defines a voicing that is present as 'a clear and balanced resonant toned voice' (2018) and Boston, drawing on Estill, alludes to a similar approach to the physiology of vocal presence, one that 'associates vocal presence with optimal vibratory conditions of vocal fold contact' (2018).

However, vocal presence can also move beyond the bounds of the individual body and physiological or psychological notions of tension and release. Oram, for example, re-posits vocal presence as a 'byproduct of an active cycle of attention and intention,' shifting between 'sensing' or 'receiving' the physicality of one's own 'awareness of feeling, thought, breath and vibration' – seen as *attention* – and a directed-ness to 'the others in the scene, the acoustic space and the audience' – defined as *intention* (2018). Such cyclical understandings of the temporality of presence begin to modulate it towards relationality, either in connection with textual and sonic material or with the given architecture, the partners and the spectators of the actor-trainee. Garvey ponders whether in fact vocal presence could be defined as 'maintaining vocal composure when in front of an audience/listener' and proceeds to offer another definition, one that foregrounds the rhythmicity of presence and its implicit mutuality: 'A speech pace which is sustainable for both speaker and, importantly, for the listener to absorb what the speaker is saying without needing to work hard, giving both speaker and listener time to breathe between thoughts or statements' (2018). In her contemplation of vocal presence, Karantonis references a phrase – possibly of Jacobean origin – that a colleague shared with her:

> "Let me hear thee so that I may see thee." [...] I tell students this because we're imbued in a visual culture and they often conceive that self-image is

purely a two-dimensional cinematic still. Whereas vocal presence is enveloping. I still think of vocal presence as a visceral immediacy.

(2018)

Reference to voicing in front of an audience engages with an understanding of voice as an in-between, as equally pertaining to the moment of production and the moment of reception. Is the trainee voicer then exclusively concerned with the moment of production? How does a trainee learn to be the primary listener of their own voice too? How do they learn to be vocally present as voicer-listeners? How can they develop a sense of sensory monitoring of their vocality as aspiring professionals? A related notion could be that of control and the question would then be reformulated: how can the trainee develop skills in controlling their voice *while* voicing? Interviewed voice practitioners generally avoid or deflect the question of control. 'I'm not sure if I do train vocal control,' Lapidge said, 'I think I try to train vocal freedom, ease and purpose' (2018). McLean replied: 'I am reticent to use the word control at all,' and further asserted: 'I believe it is focused playfulness that brings about lifeful presence' (2018). Oram was even more direct when asked how he trains vocal control in relation to vocal presence: 'I don't' (2018). According to McLean, actors 'who become obsessed with means of "controlling" their voice lose all sense of play and limit their presence entirely' (2018), while, for Karantonis,

> listening to oneself is a kind of ontological crutch and I know that classical singing teachers work against this. The voice that you hear inside your head while you are phonating is not the same voice or quality that the audience will hear.
>
> *(2018)*

Further, Garvey contends that control 'can distract the speaker from finding and maintaining a connection with what they are saying' (2018).

Having said that, Garvey equally maintains that 'it is sometimes really important for the singer to listen to their own voice, particularly for pitching and when monitoring dynamics of the melody' (2018). Does this imply, then, that not all self-listening is destructive and that only specific *types* of monitoring the voicing self – types conventionally encapsulated in the notion of 'control' – are anathema to voice training? After all, published pedagogies of the voice do encourage trainees to routinely fine-tune such listening. In the 1970s and 1980s, for example, RADA speech trainer Michael McCallion's claim that 'acute and accurate aural and sensory appreciation must be developed' (1988: 103) happily coincided with RSC voice coach Cicely Berry's assertion that 'listening accurately is one of the most important factors in using the voice fully' (1973: 123). Boston explains that although she does work against the 'self-critic activated when hearing one's "own" voice,' dismissed as 'intrusive' and 'negative,' she does not abandon listening to oneself altogether: concerted effort must be made to replace it with 'positive self-perception' instead (2018). Such an approach coincides conceptually with the scope of McLean's training, one aim of which is to 'develop a constructive relationship with listening to your own voice but by removing your ego self from the activity' (2018).

Self-listening, then, opens up the possibility of a time gap between phonating/ voicing and perceiving/hearing. It is that time gap that potentially disrupts the possibility of playful presence – particularly in so far as it provides the time/space for self-consciousness to interrupt the temporal flow of the performance or training activity. Such potential interference of the negative 'self-critic' or 'ego self' with vocal presence, the very possibility that the self-as-listener can render the present of the self-as-voicer disjointed, implies that presence in voicing is sought at the precarious juncture of two positionalities. The voicer and the listener are both singly incorporated by the trainee and, if full vocal presence involves (non-intrusive or non-egocentric) self-listening as sensitive and discerning monitoring, the aspiration that underpins the training of presence is to integrate the two perspectives so that the temporal distance between them is minimized – or, at least, is not experienced as a fundamental gap. In this sense, developing the skillset to perceive, evaluate and process auditory feedback might be key to professional voicing but presents a remarkable challenge from the perspective of embodied temporality.

This pedagogical conundrum resonates with findings in speech science and pathology.[6] As early as 1975 (S94), neurologist Barry Wyke proposed that trained voicers operate within a 'triple temporal sequence' comprised of 'prephonatory tuning' (physiological preparations prior to sounding), 'intraphonatory reflex modulation' (rapid adjustments while voicing) and 'postphonatory acoustic automonitoring' (which follows the vocal output). In this scheme, the moment of presence is either tripartite or, if actual, sounded phonation is to be taken as the sole duration and pragmatic definition of presence, the phenomenological presence of vocality is inextricably woven with its immediate pasts and futures. Voicing is irrevocably determined by vocal onset, the way the vocal musculature gets into the shape demanded by specific phonatory acts prior to their execution. Further, the monitoring and post factum perception of any voiced outcome instantly imposes readjustments and modifications to the relevant musculature.[7] This is not only configured into the new onset for a subsequent vocal gesture but also bears within it the corporal trace of the preceding voicing and its internal – both voluntary and reflex – assessment. In Husserlian terminology, the present of voicing moves beyond the immediate sensory impression of sounding to engage the *retention* of prephonatory arrangements as felt, muscular memory, alongside the anticipation of postphonatory somatic evaluation as *protention*. The voicer-listener enacts an extended vocal present. The temporal movement of this present is far from straightforwardly serial, a mere progression from onset to phonation and onwards to vocal offset. Rather, all three can be experienced as constitutive and integral components of the very act of phonation, a branching-out of the moment of voicing to encompass its approximate past and future, both now imploded, sensed and (re)trained as 'the present.'

Laryngologists D. Garfield Davies and Anthony F. Jahn have proposed a two-fold model, observing that 'the voice produced by the singer is constantly monitored in two ways: by audition and by proprioception' (2004: 10). The voicer listens to the pitch, volume and timbre of the auditory outcome through acoustic feedback from the space and, further, relies on the physical, vibratory sensation engendered by voicing within the body. The latter, proprioceptive self-experiencing of the trainee's voice is not only involved in the moment following phonation as postphonatory acoustic automonitoring (*did this feel right?*). In fact, several voice trainers emphasize the proprioceptive sensation of prephonatory onset as most crucial for monitored voicing (*if all muscles required for this specific vocal task feel right before voicing, then I need to trust that the voice produced will be the desired/intended one*). Among the six interviewees, Karantonis, rather than seeing monitoring as an activity of listening afterwards, relates vocal control to the moment of breathing, a moment *prior to* the making of sound and suggests that 'control' could be substituted by approaches to 'breath management' or 'breathing coordination': 'vocal control ultimately comes down to awareness and has to be inspired by related somatic disciplines' (2018). Somaticity is implied in Garvey's approach too: 'I do not routinely promote listening to one's voice. Rather, I invite a kinaesthetic awareness when speaking' (2018). Similarly, Professor of Music Acoustics Johan Sundberg – while concurring that voicers rely on internal and external hearing of their voice as well as physical, vibratory sensation – proposes that 'auditory feedback is not a very reliable source of information' and emphasizes kinaesthetic, 'complementary feedback signals' for controlling phonation (1987: 159–60). Voicers, 'before starting the muscular manoeuver, must "know" exactly what muscles to contract, at what moment and to what extent,' and Sunberg hypothesizes that this knowledge is muscular memory, 'probably realized by means of experience or training' (1987: 180). In the pedagogic literature, physio-vocal trainer Experience Bryon, who dedicates a large part of her methodology to the emergence of presence, goes as far as to suggest that the core preoccupation of the present-ful voicer is with the moment before presence occurs, because

> by the time any sound is produced it is really too late to "do" anything about it. […] The quality of sound […] is rather the symptom of a sort of breath dance, initiated from a centre and released through a set of controlled counterpressures in the breath-body.
>
> *(2014: 166)*

This renders the interplay of immediate vocal sensation, retention and protention even more intricate. The trainee is invited to sense the retention of vocal onset not solely as the past opening up the temporal horizon of the present of voicing but also as the protention of a future embedded in this gone-by onset, as the hope, aspiration and trust that this embodied vocal strategy will work. In other words, during the extended present of phonation, the trainee can experience the prephonatory stage simultaneously as direct past/retention (*during onset, the muscles were arranged in this specific way for me to be able to voice thus*) and as a germinal past involving the current present as a future (*during onset, the muscles were arranged in this specific way and therefore I should trust that how I am currently voicing is in accordance with what was intended*).

Whether following Wyke's tripartite template of monitored voicing (pre-, intra-, post-phonatory gestures), Davies and Jahn's binal schematization (before/proprioception and after/proprioception and audition) or Bryon's primary investment in one aspect of temporality (past/preparation) towards relinquishing the emergence of presence, the intersection of voicing and self-listening in the dual cultivation of the trainee as present voicer and monitoring listener posits *the present* as a fundamental problem for *presence*. Even if voicers are trained to 'be in the moment' or to 'achieve presence,' they can only rely on post-voicing auditory feedback or pre-voicing kinaesthetic awareness; voice perception is *always-not-yet* there or *always-already* there. Both trainers and trainees, then, have to grapple with an understanding of embodied time that simultaneously sublimates fully resonant presence and renders it intangible. How does one then train to work against (or with) the elusiveness of vocal presence? Which skillsets are required? How are they cultivated?

Timespacing vocal presence: from idiotopic endochrony to allotopic exochrony

Jane Boston asserts that an advantageous starting point for training vocal presence is breath, as 'phonation depends on the appropriate manipulation of breath pressure and its conscious application for the production of efficient soundwaves' (2018). An aim of her training approach is to

> enable students to both feel and engage with breath as a conscious activity. As conscious awareness surfaces, it is attended to in the form of a focus on muscular activities – collectively known as support – that get directed for specific performance outcomes whilst also remaining in association with breath as a source of release and ease. In combination, this creates the conditions for vocal presence as derived from the conscious awareness of unconscious life-giving forces that reveal the simultaneous paradox of control and release.
>
> *(Boston 2018)*

The underpinning impulse of the work is 'to ensure that students are able to verify their own roots to the impulse of breath and vibration in order to validate their own internal processes' (Boston 2018). Oram frames his approach in a similar way in stating that 'the work is bounded by a principle of ease and limited by a desire to avoid injury'; the trainee first learns 'to pay attention to core principles of breath, thought, feeling and vibration' and 'the training begins with listening to the self and a form of self-verbatim, which challenges the actor to translate the "everyday" self into a "theatrical everyday"' (2018). Garvey also emphasizes the significance of breath and of paying attention to it before voicing: the trainees need to 'really connect with their own breath before speaking' and identify 'the moment of "resting" before the new breath drops in' (2018). Inspired by Kristin Linklater's methodology, the first exercise Garvey proposes as aiding the cultivation of presence is for the student to approach another person and, while maintaining direct eye contact, say their name. In a similar vein, Karantonis has adapted Lee Strasberg's 'Song and Dance' exercise towards training for vocal presence:

> I ask students to chant their name and move slowly around a circle formed by their peers. The exercise is really about building a strong nerve in the face of the other (your audience) and now allowing your voice to give way in that moment.
>
> *(Karantonis 2018)*

McLean proposes a slightly different point of departure. She experiments with 'the common level of energy' in the group of trainees, uses 'harmony and dissonance in song' and facilitates a 'sense of play and dialogue' between members of the ensemble (2018). The training does not always begin from physiological principles of voice production but is 'tailored to meet bespoke aims, i.e. towards text, or to address concerns around confidence in performance, to focus on harmonizing skills, to look at extending range etc.'; key to McLean's training is

> encouraging players to see the sound as something separate to themselves [...] and to facilitate them in finding and helping create partners that can help them generate the sound that rings. This can be with an instrument, a partner, or even with dramaturgical concepts/visualizations.
>
> *(2018)*

In a comparable approach, Lapidge suggests that vocal work is always in connection to 'a partner of some kind' (2018). Further, she specifies:

> I have been working more and more with exercises that work with feedback loops, with listening to one's own voice and others' voices, including the merging of multiple voices. I have noticed that students, when asked to speak a text into a space in the room which gives them a very immediate and resonant feedback or echo, are impacted by the sound of their own voice – it can reveal itself more to them in this way. For some it makes them feel self-conscious, for others it makes them feel free from their pre-occupation of 'how does my voice sound?'
>
> *(Lapidge 2018)*

Through the above pedagogic gestures and formulations of concrete vocal strategies, two approaches to the temporality of vocal presence emerge – approaches that are both practical in their hands-on, studio-based repercussions for trainees and paradigmatic in their theoretical implications. For the first paradigm, the temporality of presence, its being-in-time, departs from the body of the trainee. The training first invites the trainee to engage with somatic adjustments related to the release of psychophysical blocks through conscious or self-aware connection to breath and easeful manipulation of the vocal anatomy. The entry point to the 'complex present of vocal presence,' as posited in the previous section, evidences kinship with Wyke's delineation: the trainee is invited to experience vocality as starting with prephonatory preparation and emanating outwards. Boston fittingly captures this movement and its ongoing anchoring in the trainee's self: 'Once a student is brought into the world of "being" in the studio in democratic ways that are student centred and non-didactic, their experience is channelled towards the generation of trust in sound-making attached to their own internal "benchmarks"' (2018). The cultivation of the trainee as voicer and listener begins with listening-in to the prephonatory internality of the self, extends into an intraphonic moment of vocal production and culminates in a postphonatory listening-out to the self in the space and with others. In some instances, the transition towards externality involves an act of announcing or narrating the self, as in the naming exercises shared by Garvey and Karantonis or the notion of 'self-verbatim' by Oram.

The second paradigm engages the trainee in the reverse temporal structuring of presence. The point of departure is a being-with-others, be they fellow trainees, aspects of the given architecture or textual and sonic scores. The originary presupposition is that the vocal self is fundamentally and *a priori* porous, therefore prephonation is imagined as a playful and dialogic – to return to McLean's wording – listening of the self in the process of co-voicing. In Lapidge's example of speaking text within an idiosyncratic acoustic, the trainee is first impacted by the voice as returned to them via the space. The echo of the voiced self – foregrounded precisely as such: a distant and acoustically mediated version of one's sound – inaugurates the coming-forth of vocal presence. Listening to one's voice means listening-with. The interrogation of the internal make-up of vocality is not avoided but emerges as an outcome in a scheme that postulates listening-out as prephonation and any physiological readjustments or moments of return to the self as postphonatory. Whereas in the first paradigm the emergence of vocal presence was initiated by the internal reorganization of the self, Lapidge foregrounds the emphasis of the second paradigm on external stimuli in proposing that 'vocal presence could be considered a continuum, something that is not fixed but which, if sought, *must respond to or be attuned to* its speaker, audience and its context. What is appropriate for the voice in any given context?' (2018; added emphasis).

In both strands of work, the emergent present of vocality entangles time and space in 'a certain timespace,' an interweaving of time and space that is both generated by each approach to voice training and enables the coming-forth of trained vocal presence in ways that go 'beyond the immediately present or presented' (Malpas 2015: 34–35). In this sense, the first paradigm advances what I understand as *idiotopic endochrony* (ἴδιος = of the self or the individual + τόπος = place, location / ἔνδον = inside, within + χρόνος = time), a positing of the internal self as the source of temporality. Phonation reverberates first in the space of internality before it reaches external spatiality. Further, the fact that the timeline of presence starts from the self makes the space of internality come forth to the consciousness of the trainee before external space is phenomenologically engaged. Several established methodologies of voice training embrace, at least tacitly, such a model: in Cicely Berry, Patsy Rodenburg or Michael McCallion's work, voicing starts with breath and, consequently, voice training starts from releasing physical tension and directing awareness to the mechanics of easeful and efficient breathing – an understanding also mirrored in the structure of their published work. This attention to internality may even take the form of locating the emergence of voicing in specific anatomical structures (for example, the diaphragm or the pelvic muscles), and the foregrounding of prephonation/ preparation may also extend the past of phonation backwards to the personal history of the trainee (who now needs to learn to get rid of its psychophysical imprint on vocal presence).

Conversely, the second paradigm is one of *allotopic exochrony* (ἄλλος = other, else + τόπος = place / ἔξω = out, outer + χρόνος = time), a conceptualization of temporality as originating elsewhere than the self.[8] Vocal presence first involves a perceptual response to others and the space, so that the vocal present as a phenomenal occurrence is launched by the appearance of externality to the voicer's consciousness before it then folds in with the sounding self. Listening-out precedes sounding or any listening-in associated with somatic reassessment, therefore rendering the emergence of vocal presence unequivocally intersubjective from the outset. Training practices linked to Grotowskian and post-Grotowskian work tend to embrace such an approach, but this model can also be found in parts of the conservatoire sector and related publications. For Evangeline Machlin, for instance, listening to others, rather than the self, was the cornerstone of her teaching. Her training always began with listening exercises, instead of breathing, because 'listening […] is the basis of all speech acquisition' and 'to retrain your voice for the stage, you must once more begin with listening' (1980: 1; see also 1–16). Recently, Dona Soto-Morettini has also based the main bulk of her voice work in a series of carefully designed listening exercises that aim at a sharp understanding of vocal style (2014: 74–146). Prephonation in such cases is reconfigured as an encounter through the senses, as the meeting point between the self-as-it-embarks-on-voicing and the acoustic qualities of spaces, the co-resonance of others or the materiality and potency of pre-existing vocal habitus (texts, genres, traditions). In Lapidge's words, 'there is value in considering how we receive the voices of others which is a part of the sum of what it means to have "vocal presence"' (2018).

The impact of each model on the training of vocal presence is significant. The temporal narrative implied in each pedagogy of vocality comes with and instils in the trainee a wider narrative of the voicing self. 'I begin voicing from my own past and physicality and then move outwards' or 'I begin by listening to the outside and then I respond in voicing' are both narratives that can move beyond ways of being-present-in-voice towards reorganizing the trainee's ontological perception of themselves. In this sense, the timespace of the 'complex present of present' is not uniformly phenomenological but always-already ideological. Individual response to the self-perception of voicing, originating either in pre- or post-phonation, is trained to become 'muscle memory' (to return to Sundberg), but this memory is not independent of the value that the trainee accords this self-listening in relation to the feedback received by others, within and outside of training. Listening to one's self, listening to one's voice and listening to one's self as the originator or recipient of voicing overlap, but are not identical. The rates and ways in which they fold into the experience of the vocal present may vary depending on the time that different narratives of the self take up in each trainee's processing of their voicing self. What is, for example, the time lapse between external and internal feedback in the timespace of presence for trainee-voicers that do not partake in the cultural dominant (in and outside the class)? How does placing voicing in the elsewhere of allotopic exochrony empower or disempower trainees who are aware that their voice may be perceived as other? And how can shifting attention away from idiotopic endochrony cultivate an activist stance if the voicing of the self is perceived as normative? In addition, the seeming linearity of each narrative ('time starts from the inside and moves to the outside' or 'time starts from the outside moves to the inside') can embed not only a timeline but, crucially, a hierarchy in the complex present of vocal presence. Being trained in perceiving one's vocal presence as originating with the self is not far from lending primary significance to that point of origination, in the same way that understanding vocal presence as departing from elsewhere may incline the trainee to prioritize their connection to externality while voicing.

However, the two temporal paradigms of emergent vocal presence, although contradictory, may not necessarily be mutually exclusive, particularly in the practices of a generation of practitioner-scholars well versed in self-reflexivity and acutely attuned to the ideological ramifications of their studio work. McLean, although primarily interested in ensemble training, is equally invested in solo work. In this context, the trainee/performer generates material, and recordings are used to help the trainee repeat, with technical precision, selected aspects of their voicing in the hope that they will later 'reignite it with the kind of presence it might have come into being with' (McLean 2018). In this case, the recording may be used to represent or substitute external stimuli, but it is a documented version of the self that is the point of interest. Lapidge, although rooting her work in what I have described as the allotopic and exochronic model, also observes that the responsiveness to impulse can become powerful when the trainee's past emerges alongside vocal presence:

Even when working with an image, or a memory or with imagination, the idea that the speaker is able to bring that into the present moment through the voice seems significant. When an actor brings to you their memory of something particular through the voice and into the present moment it can be extremely evocative.

(2018)

Boston might ground the work in the somaticity of the breath but also raises significant questions regarding training vocal presence when asking: 'who is best to verify the outcome, the individual, the voice pedagogue, or the vocal health professional?' (2018). This immediately postulates the training as a dialogic process, presents the trainee voicer as always participating in a dyad involving a listener and implies a methodological approach that does not detach exercises on vocal presence from 'the means by which to *verify* vocal presence' (Boston 2018; original emphasis). Oram also invites students to 'recognize the cultural embeddedness of the work and negotiate that dialectically' (2018). His work begins with the principles of good vocal use and an attention to breath, thought and feeling, but this is then layered further:

> We then add in the 'other'; paying attention to our partner and ourselves, we learn how the core principles shift in response to a basic relationship. We then layer in the intention of sharing that experience with the other through our voice. Then, we return to paying attention to the core principles in ourselves as we add in attention of the acoustic space and, then, the audience.
>
> *(Oram 2018)*

The timeline of presence may be launched by the self but it is then inserted into a cyclical narrative that rotates between endochrony and exochrony. Similarly, Garvey may ask trainees to speak their names as a first move towards experimenting with presence, but, immediately afterwards, she invites their partners to speak their name back to them. A second exercise sees partners exchanging ideas on how they perceive their voice but, then, each trainee has to narrate to the rest of the group not their own but their collaborator's understanding of their voice. This has the potential to destabilize the straightforward integration of selfhood and vocality, and, although grounding speaking in prephonatory breathing is paramount for Garvey, she also stresses how this should be interlinked with training the voicer to 'find and maintain a desire to share and be understood' (2018). Karantonis (2018) also invites us to think further about the allotopic and exochronic potential of vocal presence:

> The ideal vocal presence could be one that really moves audiences. Another colleague of mine once posed it as this rhetorical question: 'what do you want to leave in the ear of the audience once they have left the theatre'?

I like this as a notion of a vocal presence still nestling in the eardrum as a sympathetic vibration, going home with the audience members, until it dissipates like the moment of performance.

If – as this chapter has argued – the ephemeral and transient moment of vocal presence is experienced by the trainee simultaneously as an always-not-yet and an always-already, unfolding in a continuum between idiotopic endochrony and allotopic exochrony, then glimpses of temporal counter-narrative, such as the above, can acquire significant potency. In foregrounding that the present of vocality is both phenomenologically complex and vested with specific narratives of the self, they can open up spaces (and temporal intervals) for the trainee to embrace this complexity without succumbing to a single timeline of vocal emergence and, further, to disrupt such narratives through radical vocal praxis.

Notes

1 Sánchez-Goldberg has convincingly linked 'this body focus' with 'a progressive devaluation of language and a move towards a nonverbal idiom' (2007: 22).

2 For a recent critique of presence and embodiment in Rodenburg and other pedagogues' training, and a reconceptualization of presence through an intercultural lens, see McAllister-Viel (2018) and Thomaidis (2017: 50–57).

3 In line with the expressly praxical character of the research, the interviews quoted here represent a much larger PaR project and involvement with the practices cited; over several years, I have also observed the interviewees' practices (as participant-observer as well as workshop, performance or conference attendee) and, even, trained with some of them over longer periods of time. Similarly, all interviewees were given the option of responding to my questions in writing or verbally, some of them submitted recorded versions of their answers, and there were several follow-up discussions between us. In this sense, the written extracts are deeply embedded in ongoing, embodied vocal interchange. All interview questionnaires have been approved by the Ethics Committee of the Humanities College at the University of Exeter and relevant permissions have been sought in writing. I wish to thank and acknowledge all interviewees for their generosity and rigour.

4 Jane Boston has taught at the National Youth Theatre and RADA, is currently Principal Lecturer and Course Leader of the MA/MFA Voice Studies at Royal Central School of Speech and Drama and Head of the International Network for Voice. Deborah Garvey is Lecturer in Voice at RCSSD, having also taught for significant courses on musical theatre such as the BRIT School and London School of Music Theatre. Pamela Karantonis is Senior Lecturer in Voice at Bath Spa University (currently transitioning into a new post at Goldsmiths), holds a Ph.D. on impersonation from the University of New South Wales and co-convened the Music Theatre working group at IFTR. Lisa Lapidge holds an MA in Voice Studies from RCSSD and is currently a Lecturer on the BA Acting & Creative Practice at the University of Northampton. She was previously a core member of companies Para Active & Zecora Ura (ZU-UK). Anna-Helena McLean has taught for the BA Vocal and Choral Studies at the University of Winchester and the Royal Conservatoire of Scotland, and was a principal actor-musician with Gardzienice before establishing her company Moon Fool and developing her methodology 'Actor-Chorus Text.' Daron Oram is Senior Lecturer in Voice at RCSSD, having also taught at other major drama schools, such as East 15 and Italia Conti, and was the Head of the BA Musical Theatre at ArtsEd for six years.

5 I have argued elsewhere about the necessity of re-vocalizing academic discourse in/ about/through voice (Thomaidis 2015a) and the epistemic benefits of polyphonic writing as undercutting the

> logocentric prioritization of the written over the phonic *from within*; the personal, I – thou, perhaps less structured but not less rigorous tone of this style resists the exnomination of analytical discourse by disrupting its seeming conceptual self-sufficiency in otherwise monographic/monologic texts.
> *(Thomaidis in Karikis et al. 2016: 175; original emphasis)*

6 For thorough summaries and discussion of existing scientific research on vocal control and perception, consult Kreiman and Sidtis (2013: 57–71, 89–108) and Sundberg (1987: 157–81). My analysis resonates with Kreiman and Sidtis's inclusive understanding of control and perception: 'It is important to remember that pitch, loudness, and quality are psychological characteristics, and as such they represent the impact of physical signals on human ears' (2013: 57).

7 The cognitive time-lapse between voicing, listening to one's voice and adapting is minuscule and probably experienced as a process occurring before the voicer-listener is aware of it or acknowledges it as a delay. Specifically researching auditory feedback and pitch in singers performing melodic leaps, Sundberg writes: 'one sometimes can observe a second pitch change, typically occurring some 200 or 300 msec after the main pitch change. This leads us to postulate that the pitch change should lead to the correct target *at once*' (1987: 180; added emphasis).

8 In studies in education, Michel Alhadeff-Jones has proposed exochrony as 'a capacity to detach oneself from a familiar experience of time' (2016: 211). In proposing exochrony here, I am not concerned with experiences out of time but with experiencing time as being or emerging outside the self. Philippe Amen has used endochronie/ endochrony in literary studies to denote 'a temporality used by the writer's self (*soi-même*), a self-sufficient time, a time breaking with that of the social body' (2016; my translation). To my understanding, neither author posits the two terms in a continuum, and my argument here is emphatically concerned with timespace rather than solely time, hence my coinage of allotopic exochrony and idiotopic endochrony.

References

Alhadeff-Jones, M. (2016) *Time and the Rhythms of Emancipatory Education: Rethinking the Temporal Complexity of Self and Society*, Oxon and New York: Routledge.

Amen, P. (2016) 'Une folle liberté que je dois maîtriser pour me dire: endochronies du journal intime,' *Polysèmes*, 17. http://journals.openedition.org/polysemes/2011.

Berry, C. (1973) *Voice and the Actor*, New York: Hungry Minds.

Boston, J. (2018, 4th July) 'Interview with K. Thomaidis,' UK.

Bryon, E. (2014) *Integrative Performance Practice: Practice and Theory for the Interdisciplinary Performer*, Oxon and New York: Routledge.

Cavarero, A. (2005) *For More than One Voice: Toward a Philosophy of Vocal Expression*, trans. P.A. Kottman, Stanford, CA: Stanford University Press.

Davies, D.G. and Jahn, A.F. (2004) *Care of the Professional Voice*, London: A&C Black.

Garvey, D. (2018, 24th July) 'Interview with K. Thomaidis,' UK.

Karantonis, P. (2018, 24th July) 'Interview with K. Thomaidis,' UK.

Karikis, M., Mitchener, E., Walker, J. and Thomaidis, K. (2016) 'Voice in devising/ devising through voice: a conversation with Mikhail Karikis, Elaine Mitchener and Jessica Walker,' *Journal of Interdisciplinary Voice Studies*, 1(2): 173–82.

Kreiman, J. and Sidtis, D. (2013) *Foundations of Voice Studies: An Interdisciplinary Approach to Voice Production and Perception*, Chichester: Wiley-Balckwell.

Lapidge, L. (2018, 6th July) 'Interview with K. Thomaidis,' UK.

Machlin, E. (1980) *Speech for the Stage*, London and New York: Routledge.

Malpas, J. (2015) 'Timing space-spacing time: on transcendence, performance and play,' in Grant, S., McNeilly, J. and Veerapen, M. (eds) *Performance and Temporalisation: Time Happens*, Basingstoke: Palgrave Macmillan, 25–36.

McAllister-Viel, T. (2018) *Training Actors' Voices: Towards an Intercultural/Interdisciplinary Approach*, Oxon: Routledge.

McCallion, M. (1988) *The Voice Book*, London: Faber and Faber.

McLean, A.-H. (2018, 19th June) 'Interview with K. Thomaidis,' UK.

Oram, D. (2018, 28th June) 'Interview with K. Thomaidis,' UK.

Rodenburg, P. (2007) *Presence: How to Use Positive Energy for Success in Every Situation*, London: Michael Joseph (Penguin Books).

Sánchez-Goldberg, A. (2007) 'Altered states and subliminal stages: charting the road towards physical theatre,' in Keefe, J. and Murray, S. (eds) *Physical Theatres: A Critical Reader*, Oxon and New York: Routledge, 21–25.

Soto-Morettini, D. (2014) *Popular Singing and Style*, London: Bloomsbury.

Sundberg, J. (1987) *The Science of the Singing Voice*, DeKalb, IL: Northern Illinois University Press.

Thomaidis, K. (2015a) 'The re-vocalization of logos? Thinking, doing and disseminating voice,' in Thomaidis, K. and Macpherson, B. (eds) *Voice Studies: Critical Approaches to Process, Performance and Experience*, Oxon and New York: Routledge, 10–21.

———— (2015b) 'What is voice studies? Konstantinos Thomaidis,' in Thomaidis, K. and Macpherson, B. (eds) *Voice Studies: Critical Approaches to Process, Performance and Experience*, Oxon and New York: Routledge, 214–16.

———— (2017) *Theatre & Voice*, Basingstoke: Macmillan/Springer.

Wyke, B. (1975) 'Neuromuscular control systems in singing,' *The Journal of the Acoustical Society of America*, 58: S94.

17

REHEARSING (INTER)DISCIPLINARITY

Training, production practice and the 10,000-hour problem

Laura Vorwerg

Imagine this: you arrive on the first day of rehearsals with the feeling of dread which accompanies the dream where you are on stage, naked and cannot think of a single thing to say or do. In a few short weeks, you will be exposing yourself in a different way: you will be performing an entirely new skill, something outside of your disciplinary knowledge. You have no training in this alien discipline, yet, somehow, by the end of the rehearsal process, you will need to engage those skills in front of an audience, whose enjoyment of the work, according to Marvin Carlson (2006: 3), is predicated on their recognition of your skill.

★★★★★★

Performing is an exposing and precarious activity, and making yourself vulnerable in this way often feels, as Experience Bryon aptly puts it, 'like risking your life' (2015). This precarity is magnified when performance skills outside of those developed through rigorous training are demanded as part of a production's aesthetic or as a pragmatic solution to a core creative challenge, for example, the representation of a non-human character. Yet interdisciplinary performance practice, which has emerged in response to contemporary pluralist tastes for diverse performance aesthetics and artistic innovation, often includes the creation of a production-specific skill-base in order to meet specific creative challenges. New disciplinary skills may have to be developed quickly within the time-restricted process of rehearsal; performers can be expected to learn skills in silk climbing, puppetry and/or martial arts to supplement – or perhaps as an extension of – their own practice as actors, opera singers or dancers. Accessing another disciplinary skill-set in this way presents a temporal anomaly between the few hundred hours typically available for rehearsal and the 10,000 hours of dedicated practice necessary to master such skills, an anomaly we might refer to in this context as 'the 10,000-hour problem.' Drawing on examples from theatre and opera to consider how this temporal mismatch is resolved in practice, this essay interrogates the ways in which time restrictions influence skill acquisition in rehearsals, understood here as creative but *also as* training contexts. It also proposes possible strategies for rehearsing (inter)disciplinarity which circumvent the opposing pressures of aesthetic diversification and extended disciplinary practice.

Studies investigating skill acquisition have long established that it requires approximately 10,000 hours of dedicated practice to develop an expert level of skill. This timeframe roughly equates to three hours a day for ten years or 40 hours a week for five years. The first such study conducted by Simon and Chase (1973) focused on chess players but various studies in cognitive science have since indicated that this timeframe applies equally in any specialized disciplinary training including that of musicians, surgeons, athletes and dancers.[1] This period remains the same whether training is condensed, such as in the intense study and long hours of those in the medical profession, or is spread over the course of childhood or young-adulthood, as is common when studying ballet or a musical instrument. Neuroscientist Daniel Levitin observed that the frequency with which the figure of 10,000 hours is cited in these studies indicates that this is the requisite period required by the human body to achieve a level of mastery in any discipline in which one can be considered expert (2006: 197). Noting that there has yet to be a case of world-class expertise accomplished in less time, Levitin suggests that this phenomenon is consistent with the way in which the brain assimilates and consolidates information in neural tissue. Learning requires that new information be processed and stored as a neural trace and, whilst the time taken to consolidate information neurally varies between individuals, the strength of that memory and therefore the effectiveness of the learning experience is increased through repetition (2006: 197). The old adage that 'practice makes perfect' has within it a kernel of truth.

Richard Sennett also supports the 10,000-hour theory in his volume *The Craftsman*, noting crucially that it is the quality of the engagement or attention during training or practice that ensures development in skill- or craft-based activities. Mindless repetition does little to develop skill and time served does not necessarily equate to expertise. Expert skill development requires a quality of attention in repetition which observes and responds to tiny variations in order to refine one's engagement and, therefore, skill in that task. As Bryon has it, it is 'this *way* of *doing,* the *Practice* of the *practice*' (2014: 50; original emphasis) that demands time. Sennett borrows the term 'tacit knowledge' (2009: 50) from Michael Polanyi and uses it to refer to physical action which has become embedded corporeal knowledge.[2] Through dedicated practice, what was once a complex exchange of thoughts and physical responses, such as driving a car, working a lathe, or playing a scale, becomes seemingly instinctive tacit knowledge. Sennett argues that, *in the moment of* performance, such knowledge is flexible, responsive and adaptive. When engaged, tacit knowledge responds to shifting stimuli, utilizing skills gained through experience to adapt to minute changes in environment or to the actions of collaborators. Reaching this level of expert responsiveness, however, takes time: 10,000 hours to be roughly precise.

Whilst disciplinary training for performers may reach this figure when we include the years of practice undertaken as children and young adults prior to commencing a programme of vocational training, interdisciplinary practice which requires performers to develop new skills within the relatively brief, time-sensitive conditions of a rehearsal period does not come close to this suggested timeframe. If we budget for an optimistic four-week rehearsal period, with each week consisting of six days, each with two sessions (complying with UK industry guidelines), the total accumulated hours equal a mere 128 hours and for three weeks the total is just 96 hours. This brief calculation indicates the extent of the temporal mismatch between the development of disciplinary skill and its introduction within interdisciplinary production processes. Yet, the existence of interdisciplinary practices indicates that it is possible to bridge this gap, thereby enabling the breakdown of established disciplinary boundaries. In considering examples of interdisciplinary practice from the genres of theatre and opera, it is possible to identify three approaches which facilitate the inclusion of disparate performance skills within a single production aesthetic: *selective skill development, collaborative disciplinary integration* and *collaborative skill augmentation*. This terminology is proposed with a view to stimulate discussion around current processes and possibilities of interdisciplinary practice and as a consideration of the relationship(s) between embodied knowledge, skill and production processes.

A pragmatic approach to developing skill(s) within a reduced production timeframe is to explore only those skills necessary to meet the creative and aesthetic demands of that particular production. Such *selective skill development* makes optimal use of the time available by focusing attention around a particular skill or operation within a larger disciplinary framework. By way of example, let us consider Anthony Minghella's production of *Madame Butterfly* (Metropolitan Opera, New York, 2006, and English National Opera, 2013). Minghella's production generated plenty of column inches, many of those about Sorrow, Cio-Cio-San's child, which was, in this case, a puppet, operated by three puppeteers from Blind Summit.[3] The challenge faced by the singers playing Cio-Cio-San, Suzuki (her servant) and Lt. Pinkerton was to interact with the puppets, a skill in itself, as the illusion of life is maintained not just by the puppeteers but by anyone who performs alongside them. This is particularly crucial at moments of physical contact with a puppet as they seldom mirror the physical qualities and manoeuvrabilities of the human or animal they represent. Despite developing this puppetry skill, it is unlikely that the singers will be able to transfer their knowledge to another production. Puppetry is not commonly found in opera, nor does this experience make them puppeteers: they learned only to interact with the puppets rather than to operate them. As a process, *selective skill development* facilitates the expedient resolution of creative challenges which could potentially reduce the total hours required for rehearsal or research and development, but it does not support the individual performer as practitioner. By learning a fragment of the disciplinary skill set, the performer is potentially left exposed in the moment of performance, lacking the experiential knowledge to respond to the shifting demands and minute variations in circumstance which make each live performance different from the last. The skills developed here are selective, service a specific production and are, therefore, incomplete fragments of disciplinary knowledge. As such, their transferability from the specific circumstances of the production to another context is, at worst, impossible, at best, problematic.

A *Dog's Heart* (2010), co-produced by the ENO and De Nederlandse Opera in collaboration with Complicite and Blind Summit, also featured puppetry at its core. The production relied on the close relationship between disciplines and practitioners in the creation and realization of the title character Sharik, a stray dog living on the streets of Moscow. To successfully meet the creative challenge of presenting a canine protagonist, the tacit knowledge of the experienced puppeteers at Blind Summit, who have spent years developing and honing their skills, were brought to the heart of the production to create, direct and operate Sharik. Their expertise, alongside that of countertenor Andrew Watts and soprano Elena Vassilieva, who sang the internal and external voices of Sharik, respectively, allowed for a collaborative approach to this core creative challenge, integrating the existing disciplinary knowledge of all involved in the creation of a single character. The approach taken in this production posits a second model of interdisciplinary production practice, that of *collaborative disciplinary integration*. Practitioners with existing skill sets, developed over a significant period of time through disciplinary training and practice, are engaged collaboratively, integrating disparate disciplinary knowledge(s) to meet the creative demands of a particular piece. *Collaborative disciplinary integration* negates the need to develop physical skills quickly, and, as a process, is reliant on the *existing* training and experience of the experts involved. The interdisciplinary nature of the work is found in the engagement and interaction of those disciplines within the moment of performance.

The final model of practice, *collaborative skill augmentation*, operates by utilizing points of contact in the skill-bases of divergent disciplines. By engaging existing tacit knowledge developed over time, performers are able to expand and augment their existing embodied skill set, accessing a new discipline at a higher level and thereby reducing the amount of time required to master new skills. An example of such practice can be seen in the National Theatre's adaptation of *War Horse* (2007), where performers with experience in the disciplines of physical theatre, acrobatics, dance and puppetry were engaged to create a production-specific interdisciplinary skill-base. With expert guidance, actors and physical theatre artists developed skills in puppetry to bring to life Joey, the equine protagonist, and a myriad of other puppeteered objects and characters, including a huge tank. Augmenting skills in this manner, in order to circumvent the 10,000-hour problem, requires that points of contact between disciplines can be found. In this instance, the disciplinary practices of physical theatre and puppetry share skills in timing, rhythm, prehension, extended circles of attention or concentration, and rigorous bodily control, providing a common foundation from which to extrapolate, extend and augment the performers' skills. By engaging embodied knowledge already honed through their own dedicated disciplinary practice, artists were able to access the 'new' discipline of puppetry at a higher level and develop advanced skills as part of a time-sensitive rehearsal process. This of course does not mean that one can simply change disciplines; to suggest as much would be to devalue the skills, training and knowledge(s) of practitioners in any field. It is only through expert guidance and training, in this case led by Adrian Kohler and Basil Jones of Handspring Puppet Company, alongside the skilled bodily practice of the performers, that such skills can be introduced as part of a production process.

As interdisciplinary processes, *selective skill development*, *collaborative disciplinary integration* and *collaborative skill augmentation* all offer strategies towards circumventing the temporal mismatch found in the 10,000-hour problem. Whilst temporally bound in the present of the rehearsal period, each strategy engages with time, training and skill development differently. *Selective skill development* is pragmatic, focusing on the development of fragmentary skills possible within the strictly delineated timeframe of the rehearsal period. *Collaborative disciplinary integration* places value on the trained bodies of performers and is reliant on the time and energy invested by individuals in their own training prior to the moment of the interdisciplinary encounter. *Collaborative skill augmentation* similarly values existing tacit knowledges and utilizes them as a foundation for new skills, repurposing the hours of dedicated practice already embodied by the performers through an extended rehearsal period.[4] Although contemporary pluralist tastes continue to run in opposition to a culture which values depth of knowledge over breadth, the acquisition of additional skills continues to be a common requirement for performers. The interdisciplinary strategies examined here offer solutions to the issue of production-based skill development by either being selective, instead of expert, by collaborating to integrate divergent skills or by building on existing tacit knowledge. For expert skill, it seems we always need 10,000 hours of training, but it is how we choose to engage with that skill, and with the skills of others, that opens the door to interdisciplinarity.

Notes

1 Studies indicating parallel timeframes for high-level performance in arts, sports or science were conducted by J. R. Hayes (1981) and B. S. Bloom (1985), followed by a study by K. A. Ericsson and R. J. Crutcher (1990), which found consistent support for the suggested time frame of 10,000 hours or 10 years in a range of studies (all studies referenced in Ericsson and Smith 1991: 5-7).

2 For a detailed consideration of embodied knowledge and interdisciplinary practice, see Vorwerg (2018).

3 Other puppets in the production included servants and a dream version of Cio-Cio-San, although none generated the same level of interest as Sorrow.

4 It took seven weeks of rehearsal, an additional two weeks for the puppeteers, and several research and development periods, to create *War Horse*.

References

Bryon, E. (2014) *Integrative Performance: Practice and Theory for the Interdisciplinary Performer*, London: Routledge.

——— (2015, 23–25 May) 'Integrative Performance Practice Workshop,' London.

Carlson, M. (2006) *Performance: A Critical Introduction*, London: Routledge.

Chase, W.G. and Simon, H.A. (1973) 'Perception in chess,' *Cognitive Psychology*, 4: 55–81.

Ericsson, K.A. and Smith, J. (eds) (1991) *Toward a General Theory of Expertise: Prospects and Limits*, Cambridge: Cambridge University Press.

Levitin, D.J. (2006) *This is Your Brain on Music*, London: Atlantic.

Sennett, R. (2009) *The Craftsman*, London: Penguin.

Vorwerg, L. (2018) 'Embodied knowledges: interdisciplinarity and collaborative skill augmentation in War Horse,' in Aquilina, S. and Sarco-Thomas, M. (eds) *Interdisciplinarity in the Performing Arts: Contemporary Perspectives*, Msida: Malta University Press, 41–59.

18

BEYOND THE 'TIME CAPSULE'

Recreating Korean narrative temporalities in *pansori* singing

Chan E. Park

A folk music tradition is deeply connected to historical and ethnic memories and practices, yet its exterior is largely nonresponsive to the time's call. In terms of pedagogy, performance and reception, narrative songs from earlier eras pose a unique challenge: unlike popular ballads ubiquitously available and acceptable, the narrative songs from bygone eras and less frequented places must first be uncovered from the antiquated and unfamiliar exterior. *Pansori*, the genre of Korean traditional sung narrative, presents a noteworthy example of restoration in tandem with reinvention. To describe *pansori*'s cross-temporal complexity, this essay indexes its history, textual and musical formation and innovation, orality and transmission, and the perspectives of singers, audiences, and learners.

Pansori in the 1970s

In 20th-century Korea, the storysinging tradition known as *pansori* was largely shunned from the mainstream for its premodern outlook associated with negative ethnic memory: in the Confucian monarchic caste system prevalent throughout Korean history, performances derived from indigenous rituals of healing were marginalized as unsavoury acts. The practitioners and learners were almost entirely from the Jeolla regions and affiliated with Korean folk ritual or the entertainment profession. This was the reality when, in summer 1974, I met Kim Kyeonghui, a former all-female *changgeuk* (multi-singer operatic *pansori*) star singer. Kim was known for her impersonation of male characters in her vocal music. My month-long visit, during which she taught me two songs, initiated me to an art form that was virtually unknown to the Westernized urban culture in which I grew up. Striving to double her masculine husky voice phrase by phrase,

I was transported out of time. Why had I never heard this sound and songs before, and how much of Korea did I actually know? Almost half a century later, *pansori* singing continues to be a channel of fresh discovery for me: as a singer, teacher and learner.

Pansori in the 19th century

As a narrative performance risen to popularity in the 19th century and included in the national registry of cultural assets in the mid-20th century, *pansori* oscillates between preservation and rediscovery. Between the need for safeguarding traditional icons and each era's demand for reinvention, *pansori* singing has an ironic relationship with time. Drawing from indigenous ritual and folk musical and narrative aesthetics and textured in folk rhythmic and vocal stylistics, it came by way of telling or retelling popular stories of the time. The 19th century was its heyday; schools of singing and stylistics were identified around distinguished master singers competing for stardom and patronage. This was when the existing repertoires were trimmed to the Five Repertoires, the five classical stories and their sung narratives canonically represented in the *pansori* tradition, to align with Confucian teachings of the five cardinal virtues.[1] The narrative contents were given a facelift with Confucian morality as a way to please the upper-class patrons and fans, but this failed to shake the foundation of *pansori*: the ordinary people's worldview and grassroots expression. Without significant change since, the *pansori* left to us is indeed a time capsule rich with the cultures of 19th-century Korean storytelling.

Spatio-temporality of *pansori*

How does spatiality interact with the temporality of *pansori*? An answer may be apparent in the staging of Korean theatrical activity, which mostly comprised of outdoor events. Major community events like mask dance-drama or *pungmul* percussion and variety acts were staged in communal gathering places. Family healing rituals or chamber entertainment took place in the host's *maru* (roofed and half-enclosed parlour connecting the interior traffic, continuing to the courtyard below). In such spatial interaction, Korean theatre had developed as context-sensitive and mobile. *Pansori*, too, was sung in the open on a straw mat demarcating the area for singer and drummer framed by seated or standing audiences. To meet the challenges of outdoor singing without amplification for long hours, singers practised breathing and other mind-body exercises to strengthen their abdominal and vocal strength: against the deafening waterfall, for increasing volume, or the echo of silence in a cave, for a microtonal sounding board. The spatiality of *pansori* singing has been shifting towards indoor architectures and amplification technology, in turn shifting the culture of discipline and practice.

Pansori in the 20th century

In the waning years of Joseon dynasty, Emperor Gojong (r. 1863–1907) mandated the construction of a modern theatre building in his palace. Here, the singers of distinction led the task of modernizing Korean drama, by extrapolating dialogues and actions from the songs, adding limited elements of story-enacting and dividing roles among multiple singers. The effort of dramatization catalyzed a new musico-theatrical genre, *changgeuk* ('sung drama'), presently housed in the National Theater and other government-sponsored centres. *Pansori* during the 20th century was swiftly pushed to the margins by music, theatre, film, and storytelling emulating Western arts. By the time it was reclaimed as an intangible Korean cultural asset in 1964, *pansori* had nearly disappeared into obscurity. Its performative existence has since been sustained by systemic preservation and protection, including schools or other training structures. *Pansori* is a treasure according to national distinction, but it has lost favour with popular audiences in Korea.

Delivering musical literacy

Ideally, in musical performance, the presence of mind and voice, content and delivery, form one flow from start to finish. A steady flow through the labyrinth of the wayward and unpredictable mind is no easy task. As a product of the composite musical-literary culture of premodern Korean storytelling, the text of *pansori* frequently knots into baroque displays of poetic or historical erudition. While the basic storylines adopt fictional and historical repertoires, the detailed content is dense with esoteric literacy and historical knowledge few experts readily grasp. *Pansori* songs are encyclopedic catalogues of pre-20th-century Korea, from the sundry and mundane to the essential, anything of cultural or material curiosity to Koreans of that time. The narratives include varieties of cuisine, housing and architecture, formal and informal clothing, dry goods, labours and chores, officials and their positions, ceremonies, medicinal herbs, acupuncture, astrological signs, birds, beasts, fishery, trees, flowers, and more. If trainees dedicated themselves to studying every word of *pansori* texts, they could also be virtual walking dictionaries of premodern Korean civilization.

Introduced below is a passage from *Beompijungnyu*, 'There in the middle of the sea.'[2] The song is a musical masterpiece, but its lyric is an obstacle to the journey of the mind:

> At the Bonghwangdae pavilion,[3]
> The Samsan mountains[4] are shrouded in clouds but at the top,
> the two waters of Isu divide at the White Heron Islet[5]
> where Taebaek roamed.
> Reaching the Shimyang River,[6]
> Since the departure of Paek Nakcheon[7]
> The sound of pipa is no more,[8] and would I ever skip the Jeokpyeok River?!

The irony is that the song conjures powerful nostalgia while the all-too-frequent appearance of unfamiliar persons and places reels you into disengagement. The study of who everyone is and what connection they have with the places in the song is not nearly enough to maintain my focus on the lyric, and my plan is to go and 'feel' these places. As audience members cannot be expected to study and tour these places for fuller reception, I believe it is the responsibility of the singers to add conviction to their singing with as much knowledge and feeling as possible. So long as a singer continues singing without finding out what they are – and a surprising majority does not – all that amazing history will remain an enigmatic hocus-pocus with pleasing sonic textures. It is one thing to discuss mental concentration in singing and listening, but, from the perspective of reading and literacy, I am interested in finding out more about the level of comprehension of those members of 19th-century upper class at whose whim the text was revised and elevated: were they standardly able to identify these dense literary references borrowed for the *pansori* text? Or were they, too, feeling distanced from such already antiquating knowledge?

Text, music, orality

Narrative singing may be described as a tapestry of text and music where the quality of weaving is enhanced by mental concentration. The key question is whether the mind is steadfast on the storytelling or frequently wandering. The singer's mind strives to stay within the radius of performative truth by doing its best to mean what he sings and sing what he means. *Pansori* singing is a different sort of textile, however, in that warp and weft are not separate but one combined thread that takes years and decades of mnemonic training to produce. Unlike the reproduction of songs from sheet music, *pansori* is orally transmitted phrase by phrase, song after song, linearly along the storyline. Effective notational systems had been in use in Korean music from the ancient times, but mostly in court music.[9] In modern Korea, the Western staff system became the standard musical literacy in education and industry. The transcription of *pansori* into staff notation is now established as a graduate requirement for Korean traditional music majors, but I have yet to encounter one who uses it in training. Staff notation 'can display the pitches and time values quite in detail, it does not display enough other elements to express sounds' (Kim 2010: 212). Notwithstanding its many useful built-in features, staff notation lacks the function for the typically curvilineal movements of *pansori* singing so that such reproduction sounds robotic or caricatural. With *hangeul* (Korean script) for textual transcription in the 20th century and the later addition of recording technology, the traditional aural–oral method continues as the most efficient so far.

Text as storyworld

Pansori narrative in the 19th century was in a process of change and transformation: texts were continually being revised. Shin Jaehyo (1812–1884) of Gochang in the South was a lettered man keen on promoting singers and improving texts. In *Gwangdaega* (*Song of the Singer*), he lists appearance, voice, gesture, and text as the four prerequisites of a successful career in singing. Shin's work would not have come to fruition without those singers that met his colourful literacy with their musical prowess, and the songs performed by the singers were in a sense Shin's literary debut. In view of their collaboration, the textual development of *pansori* was towards a standard of erudition for patrons and high-class listeners. The text holds a similarly canonical status for most performers today. In general, creating or revising lyrics is generously accepted as a welcome gesture of innovation, but only a few venture outside the Five Narratives. Singers may feel insecure about any modification or embellishments to songs that are generations senior to themselves, or about adding original compositions to the genre. It can hardly be that people of today are musically less apt than the *pansori* singer-composers of the past. Rather, they are alienated from the temporality of *pansori*'s productive days. Instead of letting it to rest, we emulate it as the absolute virtue. Secondly, there exists such an overwhelming volume to learn – about 20 straight hours of singing if you do all five narratives – that most learners, myself included, find one lifetime not nearly enough to cover it, even just perfunctorily.

Towards personal discovery

It was Master Chung Kwonjin (1927–1986) who thankfully gave me the fundamentals of the theory and practice of *pansori* singing from 1976 until his passing a decade later.[10] Today, I continue training with a set of my teacher's recordings, and the thoughts and ideas from learning and practice substantiate my written research. I have taken part in several theatrical or musical productions of *pansori* as innovative adaptation, but my sense of innovation is discovery in my teacher's recorded voice: if you can do a vocal doubling of a phrase you could not do yesterday, that is innovation for me. By engaging this partial archive of the work of an intangible cultural asset, I am able to renew my affiliations, albeit in a mediated way, with a *pansori* community, past, present and future. The conversation between local experience and a canon of nationalized cultural text allows me to make independent discovery of new transnational possibilities, but ones that I hope are legible to fellow *pansori* singers and scholars. To communicate with English-speaking audiences, for example, I launched a bilingual interpretive *pansori* alternating English spoken passages and Korean sung passages (Park 2003: 245–72). Unable to readily find drum accompanists in the American Midwest, I started a seated *pansori* where the singer accompanies himself; in the comfort of a seated position, *pansori* singing is more storytelling and interpretation than theatrical enactment (Figure 18.1).

Without necessarily following fusion or other poststructuralist trends – the alleged 'call of our time' – studying the text and singing from the Five Narratives

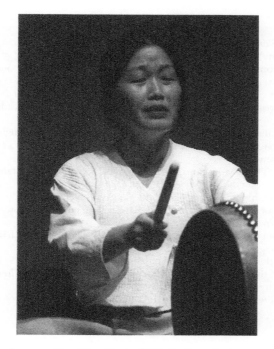

FIGURE 18.1 A solo *pansori* by Chan Park, 2000 © Chan Park.

can be a lifetime of joy. They offer effective lessons in bygone eras and allegorical forewarnings of what is yet to come. While close study of the text is not in general a prerequisite of *pansori* training, doing so can only enhance the sung performance of it. If nothing else, it will increase the level of conviction in the singing voice.

Conclusion

Closer reading and listening of the text breathe new life into *pansori* beyond its politicized and static function as icon. Closer understanding of the text forms an important bridge between the *pansori* past and the *pansori* present. In the end, *pansori* cannot be anything other than the best of what your voice and consciousness jointly produce based on your familiarity with text, language and music. A return to its basic components shows that *pansori* entails a complex temporality: convergences and divergences made out of time emerge as the pre-modern, modern, and transnational contexts are all apparent in the performance and transmission of *pansori* today. In the final analysis, singing *pansori* is a two-step mental exercise: empty the mind, and fill it with an enhanced flow of narrative reality.

Notes

1 *The Song of Shim Cheong* (for teaching filial piety), *The Song of Chunhyang* (to promote wifely chastity), *The Song of Heungbo* (brotherly love), *The Song of the Water Palace* (allegorical comedy of error about loyalty to your master) and *The Song of the Red Cliff* (gentlemanly code of repaying moral debts).
2 From *Pansori Sugungga, 'Song of the Water Palace': The Canonical Narrative as Retold by Chung Kwonjin*, translation and introduction by Chan E. Park (draft prepared for publication).
3 'Phoenix Pavilion,' on the Bonghwang Mountain in the Gangnyeongbu (江寧府, 南京) of Gangsoseong (江蘇省). These and the subsequent Chinese names are Romanized in Korean phonetics.
4 Samsan, the 'Three Mountains,' are Hwangsan, Ryeosan and Antangsan.
5 From the poem by the Tang poet Yi Baek (李白).
6 Shenyang (in Chinese) River, branch of Yangtse River.
7 Given name for Baek Geoi (白居易, 772–846), a Tang poet who wrote the 612-character poem 'The pipa song' (琵琶行).
8 Banished from his home in the Capital, one day Baek heard a familiar home-style *pipa* played by a vagrant woman.
9 Examples include: *Yukpo*, instrumental onomatopoetic mnemonics; *Yulchabo* utilizing the names of the twelve pitches (*yul*); mensural notation termed *Jeongganbo*, credited to King Sejong (1397–1450).
10 Virtuoso of the *Gangsanche Poseong* singing style, designated as Preserver in 1964.

References

Kim, J.-A. (2010) 'The musical notations of Korea and Europe,' in Hwang, J.-Y., Kim, J.-A. and Lee, Y.-S. (eds) *Musical Notations of Korea*, Seoul: National Gugak Center, 193–218.
Park, C.E. (2003) *Voices from the Straw Mat: Toward an Ethnography of Korean Story Singing*, Honolulu, HI: University of Hawai'i Press.

SECTION VI

From time to times

Expansive temporalities

19

SIMULTANEITY AND ASYNCHRONICITY IN PERFORMER TRAINING

A case study of Massive Open Online Courses as training tools

Jonathan Pitches

Context

Training is moving online. From fire safety to DIY computer-building, from salsa moves to film-making, core skills are being compartmentalized, digitized and disseminated in a host of online environments. The numbers associated with this trend are staggering and rising exponentially, along with the platforms designed to deliver such training (though YouTube remains the standout source for non-specialists looking for quick fixes).[1] Massive Open Online Courses or MOOCs – short, free-to-access units of learning delivered entirely online – are a more specialist subset of the YouTube training phenomenon and appear on popular platforms such as Coursera, EDx and FutureLearn providing organized 'learning journeys' for learners all over the world.[2]

MOOCs are particularly interesting in terms of their organization of time. Inventor of the term and an early innovator in MOOCs, Dave Cormier, suggests that one of the key oppositions produced by these courses is the tension between their eventness and the fact that they endure in perpetuity, contributing to a digital student's 'lifelong learning' (2010). Using this seeming paradox as a starting point, this chapter will outline how time is uniquely organized in digital performer training and assess what, if any, potential advantages there are to its mix of synchronous and asynchronous modes of learning. I will draw on relevant testimony from students studying on a three-week MOOC, *Physical Theatre: Meyerhold's Biomechanics*, delivered on the FutureLearn platform in 2014, 2015 and again in 2018.[3] From the perspective of Lead Educator, I will outline the range of temporal dimensions encountered in MOOC education, analyse the specific temporal decisions made in the design of the MOOC and, by way of conclusion, evaluate what justification there may be in the claim that performer training will not survive in any guise of inclusiveness unless it diversifies its infrastructure and fully embraces the rise of digital culture. In this final section, Tapscott's 'Generation next' (Tapscott, 2009) and Jan Van Dijk's work on what he calls the 'network society' (Van Dijk, 2012) are used to imagine a new generation of learners, looking for collaboration and autonomy in the context of a learning environment which seems relentlessly to be speeding up.

Temporal complexity in online performer training

Cormier's assessment that MOOCs are both eventful and enduring, mixing a momentary sense of community and liveness with a longitudinal but disconnected experience is one of a number of temporal idiosyncrasies associated with Massive Open Online learning, brought particularly into focus when considering MOOCs' capacity to deliver digital training[4] online, in comparison to embodied experiences in the studio. Of course, many training regimes rely on the residue of other documents to continue to enrich participants' learning beyond the face-to-face encounter: notebooks, both published and personal, image banks and photo archives, blogs and anecdotal records. But the means by which training endures in the Massive Online Learning environment are palpably different to these more familiar forms. How, then, is time organized in digital performer training? And are there any potential advantages to its organization, viewed alongside studio training?

There are several parallel dimensions of time in MOOC learning, which coexist to form a unique experience for teacher and student. These might be summarized thus:

1. The historical content of the MOOC itself – in this case, Meyerhold's timeline.
2. Time as it is constructed within the MOOC platform (e.g. FutureLearn).
3. Time as it is designed by the educator (including attempts to improve user engagement to encourage longer time online).
4. Time as it experienced by the teacher and moderators during the MOOC.
5. Time as it experienced by the participants during the MOOC, within and beyond the MOOC itself.
6. The differing time zones of the participants.
7. The differing ages, backgrounds and trainings of the participants.
8. Time as it is experienced after the MOOC finishes.

In this chapter, I will consider points 1–3 in brief for clarity's sake but will focus in the main on points 4–7, concluding with some consideration of potential future developments in an attempt to exemplify point 8.

Let me begin with perhaps the most conventional dimension of time: that is the history of the practitioner in question, Vsevolod Meyerhold (1874–1940). This was communicated in diagrammatic terms as a timeline set up as a contextual exercise for participants. Learners were introduced to some of the notable

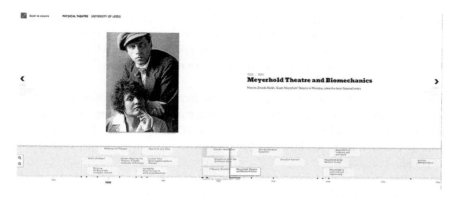

FIGURE 19.1   Meyerhold Interactive timeline, Step 1.5 on the FutureLearn Platform.

dates related to Meyerhold's history from birth to violent death, a linear history arranged in a horizontal format which could be navigated by clicking on the timeline itself (Figure 19.1).

Whilst this was not an interactive exercise, as there was no opportunity to add to the timeline itself, what was gained in using this format was a simplicity of message and an at-a-glance view of a complex period in history, including two political revolutions and several more cultural upheavals. What was lost, though, was the sense of time as layered and multi-perspectival, a historiographical view of the past which was reflected elsewhere in the MOOC's approach to Meyerhold's practice, for instance in the 'How to ask questions of a training exercise' (Step 1.10) and the 'Critical approaches to theatre history' (Step 1.4). In the former Step, an animated version of the *étude* The Slap was shown for the first time and learners were invited to construct ten questions interrogating the exercise and its place in time. This produced hundreds of responses from participants wanting to ask more of the *étude* and to problematize its context. One verbatim example from learner 'AT' gives a flavour of the kinds of comments produced by this Step:

1. Who thought of this exercise and in what context? (Is it possible to find out such an information concerning the context where this exercise was created in?)
2. In what "sets" can we divide the movements of this exercise and why some of the sets are repeated?
3. What is the purpose of this exercise?
4. From where did the creator of this exercise was influenced?
5. Where should we apply this exercise and why?
6. Do the actors have to do a specific choreography or are they taking some general instructions and are able to improvise in this?
7. From which source is this exercise comes to us today? (Historically, I mean. How credible is this source? Is it possible to have been changed during the years? Is it possible to have been misunderstood at some point?)

8. Is the slap real? How do actors feel about it? Doesn't it bother them? Is it supposed to raise feelings or is it a method to learn to keep self-control?
9. Do actors have instructions to mirror the rythm [sic] of each other?
10. What instructions you give to the actors to do this exercise?[5]

After proposing ten questions, participants then spent time answering others' questions, so there was a healthy mix of interrogative and responsive enquiry and an emergent culture of co-mentoring. Reflecting on the 2018 run of the course, DB characterized how this felt as a learner, focusing on the experiencing of time:

> I crammed in the last two weeks before the course was taken off FutureLearn. Despite this, my learning didn't feel rushed and I got a lot out of the course. I also did still feel part of the community which was very motivating and I felt free to ask questions and add to existing discussions. To my happy surprise, others, including you, were still responsive to my comments even after the conversations had long past moved on. I was very grateful for this.[6]

DB's testimony makes clear how at the level of platform design MOOC experiences are distinguished from other online teaching materials in the way in which they are time-limited in their delivery; this contributes to the 'eventness' Cormier refers to in his definition. MOOCs are normally anywhere between two and eight weeks in duration, have a specific start- and end-date and align content carefully with each week. In some platforms, this content is no longer available for scrutiny after the designated time of the course; in others, the materials are available indefinitely – to review, download, rehash and reuse without restriction.[7] There is a very real sense of a 'first day' on the course – for teacher and learner – and conversely of leaving at the end of the allotted weeks, even if the course in some cases can be reviewed by an individual for as long as they want. In pedagogical terms, the time-limited delivery of the course, allows for students to have a level of parallel experience, building to the same goals at the end of each week and opening up conversations about the same learning materials in the comment threads alongside teaching materials (Figure 19.2).

Each course is broken down into weeks and each week is broken down into 'Steps' that are completed by students before moving to the next. For instance, in the first week of the *Physical Theatre* course, there are 17 steps, broken down into four main activities: (1) Actor training in context, (2) What is biomechanics? (3) The *études* and (4) Preparation for practical activities, followed by a summative test. The majority of students follow this timetable as the opportunity to share ideas and comments in parallel with others is highly valued. The end of a week, then, becomes a kind of shared event and as in this course there was a shift from theoretical and historical materials in Week One to practical

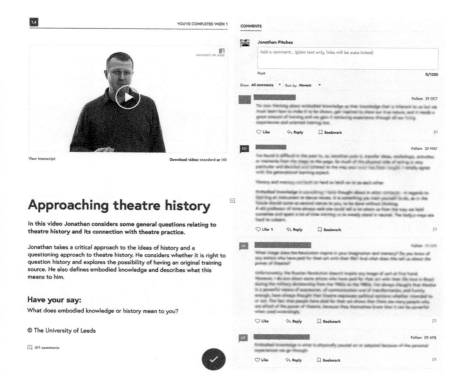

FIGURE 19.2 Comment threads alongside a video tutorial on the FutureLearn Platform.

examination of the *études* via video tutorial in Week Two, there was a particular sense of moment:

GG: Off to the garden shed now with my torch to find a stick!
SH: All very exciting. It fills me with ideas. And now, where can I get that stick?
OS: inspiring first week looking forward to practicals of week two!

Similar expectancy (and a little apprehension) characterized many of the comments at the end of the second week – 'AL: I AM VERY NERVOUS ABOUT FILMING MYSELF DOING ANY OF THE WORK!' – before, in the first part of Week Three, students were asked to share their own self-generated documents of embodying the biomechanical *étude*, the Slap, in a Facebook event, either in prose, stills or video. Students were encouraged to find for themselves an appropriate means to document their training and if writing, photography or video did not appeal, to watch others' work and comment on it. There was a palpable sense of expectation (some called it 'bravery') in this period as the participants sought to make material sense of the training of the week. Inevitably

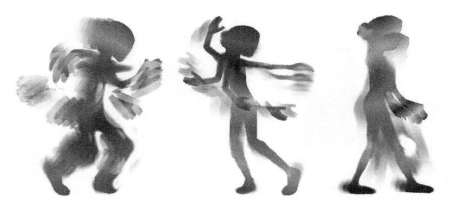

FIGURE 19.3 Participant response to Meyerhold MOOC, experience of practice.

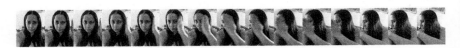

FIGURE 19.4 Participant response to Meyerhold MOOC, experience of practice.

the task of objective documentation was not always rigidly adhered to and some of the most interesting responses were produced by students working beyond the three suggested forms. LHJ's artwork[8] exemplifies this (Figure 19.3).

And JM's imaginative montage was similarly thought-provoking[9] (Figure 19.4).

Whilst the number of registered students who were prepared to expose themselves to the rest of the group just days into a training regime was a small fraction of the total (approximately 100 from 7,000 over the first two courses), these documents provided evidence of student engagement right across the world – Australia, South and North America, Europe and Asia – and constituted important primary materials for students who were still practicing the *études* but were not prepared or interested to share them. Responding to drop-off data, when students left the course or stopped commenting, the second run of this course in 2015 allowed for a longer period of embodiment and carried over the documentation of the *études* into the final week. We also trimmed back a number of the steps, so that additional theoretical and video material was categorized as 'see also' rather than mandatory. Returning learners (those coming back in week two) went up by over a hundred.[10]

For these students, the temporal experience of this MOOC was fundamentally linear and incremental as they 'bonded' as a cohort and progressed through together, step by step. For the educator and for the supporting moderating team, responding on the comment threads, the feeling was expressly *non*-linear – jumping backwards and forwards across the different activities (and weeks) to ensure that the educators' voices were present in the threads consistently, something again which was highly valued in the summative feedback. With students in different time zones moving onto the platform at different times of the day, there was no predicting when students would peak in their activity, although there were hot spots at the end of each GMT day, reflecting the number of UK-based students (43%).

Looking deeper at the evidence, though, suggests that this sharp distinction between the students' and educator's time-experience was not always backed up by the student behaviour in the comment threads. In fact, as one might flick through activity on the newsfeed in Facebook, students often moved forwards and back through the course, not so much to resist the inherent linearity of its design but to read and absorb fellow learners' comments over time – and to check if their own statements had had any replies:

JL: This is just a wonderful way to study. It's great to know the course is moving forwards, as it provides motivation to keep up, but you have the freedom to re-watch segments or read the comments and insights that are continually being added. Thank you to everyone that is contributing their thoughts so openly in these forums – I'm really enjoying hearing the perspectives of such a diverse group of people.

TG: This course has been a positive and rewarding undertaking. I continue to go back to reading various discussions as they keep growing! Fitting it in at the start of the school year has meant I've not engaged in the discussion as fully as I would have liked, but have really appreciated reading through the range of views from all the participants.

In addition to this toing and froing, a significant number of participants comment on the simultaneity of their time outside of the MOOC – time spent in their real lives or on other MOOCs. Students report catching up on the practice, after pressures at work or home, or committing to too many other free and easy to access courses:

MM: Next week: week 2 of Biometrics [sic] and week 1 of Film making. A balancing act with the rest of my activities. Bring it on! This has been so informative and enjoyable. Thank you.

DE: I am in the same boat, so I have worked my way through Week 2 of Biomechanics already (shhh)

GB: I am somehow juggling 4 of these classes at once. What was I thinking?

This is perhaps not entirely different from face-to-face training, but, as the timing and the space for the practice itself is given over to the student, the blurring of social, professional and educational life is exacerbated in the MOOC sphere. This clashing of different lives is further intensified by the mode of access to MOOCs, predominantly through the mobile technology of smart phones and tablets, used for other things such as work and socialising – strong evidence of so-called 'convergence' (Van Dijk 2012: 54–6).[11]

Just as these parallelisms were the lived experience for learners, so too were they for the educators. Without a doubt, MOOC teaching adds another layer of complexity to one's life during the weeks of delivery. As it is possible to facilitate learning in unlikely circumstances – whilst on the train, punctuating cooking in the evening or on a weekend walk – it is tempting to consider practicing a 24/7-style pedagogy whilst the MOOC is running. But in truth, the most sustainable way to engage with a cohort of many thousands of students was to dedicate a period each day to engage more deeply with the comment threads. This often meant looking up sources and refreshing my own memory in relation to historical content. It sometimes led to me performing parts of the *étude* in my own study-studio, to 'feel through' the practical issues students were experiencing – relating to balance or rhythm for instance – before narrating these back on the comment threads. It also tied me closely to the same events students were anticipating and precipitated similar levels of anxiety and self-exposure. Will anyone respond to the challenge of embodying a complicated physical *étude* after just two weeks training? How will the subtleties and individualities of biomechanics be communicated by an animated avatar? What happens if someone throws their exercise stick through the kitchen window? These are similar feelings to those experienced in a conventional teaching and learning relationship but heightened by the absence of direct visual and physical feedback from students in the same room.

Summary

The temporal idiosyncrasies of digital training are multiple and complex but there are a number of characteristics which are identifiable. First, learners do tend to move through the training incrementally and respect the temporal markers set by the educator through the design of the course and its implementation on the platform. Indeed, this is a key factor in generating a sense of community. Second, and despite this respect for the learning journey, learners value the opportunity to return to and review exercises at different times, moving backwards and forwards during the course and extending their engagement beyond what they themselves have set as their designated time online. Third, despite the absence of a shared practice in a shared space, there is a powerful sense of collective work enhanced by the common goals, the sharing of experiences and the uploading of user-generated content. This sense of moment is also experienced by the educators. Fourth, for an educator or performer trainer, there is a very unfamiliar ceding of control: no hands-on instruction, no collective control of the micro-rhythms of learning, less opportunity to individualize experiences and a non-linearity to the production of feedback; this is an unsettling but also levelling experience. Fifth, comments made by the tutor are archived and remain visible for all the tutees, flattening out some of the unforeseen hierarchies that can exist in the studio and allowing for longitudinal reflection from both student and trainer.

It is important to recognize that the data used here has an innate bias, as it is generated by self-selecting students, with a predisposition to be positive; those learners who didn't approve either left or did not comment. The experiences documented in this chapter nevertheless constitute food for thought beyond this case study and in the context of the growing online presence of training materials. What implications are there for performer training in this study and what role does the shifting temporality of the digital environment play in them?

To start to answer these questions I quote at length below from a participant's course summary, which echoes many of the themes of this chapter: non-linear learning time, convergence, the relationship between media and learning styles and the preponderance of studio hierarchies:

JGR: Really thoroughly enjoyed course, and found it a great way to be introduced to Biomechanics. In terms of using an online environment for physical actor training, it was a very positive experience, in some ways more positive than learning such skills in a studio environment. At home on my own, I really felt I was in a safe space to try the physical activities as many times as I wanted, without feeling stupid in front of others. This gave me time to really get comfortable with the exercises in a way which I wouldn't have done in a group.

I also felt in the comments, we heard voices that would sometimes stay quiet in a rehearsal room, where in my experience the most confident and the most physically able would be the most vocal during such exercises. Here we had people saying "I really struggled with that," "I was struggling but then I did this which helped me to get it," etc. As a fellow learner, these voices were really valuable. It was very helpful that the learning was cut up into sizeable chunks, including the panel discussion. The varied use of video, writing and activities was also very good. This was a very pleasant way to learn, creating a balance between active and passive learning. It proved far superior to my experience of "Teach Yourself" books, for example.

These words are clearly from a satisfied individual – though they are not uncharacteristic of the tone expressed at the end of the course. As a biomechanics practitioner, steeped in the culture of a collective workshop following a master tutor (in my case, Alexei Levinsky[12]), they nevertheless came as a surprise. JGR does not focus on the lack of direct person–person contact in the training (a significant concern for me as educator). Instead, s/he raises an often unspoken and fundamentally ethical point about the power dynamics of a studio–workshop suggesting that the digital format of training might go some way to levelling deeply ingrained hierarchies, giving voice to those who might otherwise self-censor or be overlooked. This flipped sense of power relations is created by many things – the domestic familiarity of the learning environment, the sense of agency created by being in control of the learning and of what is offered back to the group, to name two. But with our focus here on the temporal, it is worth considering how time plays a part in this democratising of the workshop experience. JGR, like many of his/her peers on the course, valued the absence of direct scrutiny so typical of performer training regimes based in studios. Instead of the pressure to absorb and embody techniques in the moment, the platform's support of *asynchronous* learning was a real boon for this student. It is seen as a form of inclusive learning, where the scope to process discoveries in *one's own time* is beneficial.

DB, an educator and practitioner, extended this idea of inclusivity in his/her reflection on the latest run of the course:

> This style of transmission is so accessible to multiple learning styles which is fantastic. Students have visuals of the entire arc of each exercise; they have visuals of information as well as hearing all of this from you; they have kinaesthetic learning in manoeuvring through these exercises themselves. The videos were short, which is great for those of us who can't focus for too long. We could see you talking and had the option to close captions, which is great for those of us who need to see lips move to understand what you're saying, and those of us with hearing impairments.[13]

Many of these adjustments for diverse learning styles and needs are not possible in the direct, one-to-one contract of a workshop session (although they may be wrapped around such sessions if a tutor uses a Virtual Learning Environment).[14] MOOC education on the other hand is designed to address these from conception to delivery.

Conclusion

Thinking beyond the specifics of the Massive Open Online community, I suggested in my introduction that performer *training* may not survive in any guise of inclusiveness unless it diversifies its infrastructure and fully embraces the rise of digital culture. To consider this position in a little more detail, I draw here on two critics, Jan Van Dijk and Don Tapscott, both of whom at their respective moments in the present, have tried to capture future advances in developed countries in relation to digital culture. For Van Dijk the future suggests '*a complete integration of online and offline types of communication,*' with '*practices of sharing* cultural forms' most prominent in young people (2012: 222, emphases in original). For Tapscott, the 'Net Generation' (born 1977–1997) and 'Generation next' (born 1998–present) are 'forcing a change in the model of pedagogy, from a teacher-focused approach based on instruction to a student-focused model based on collaboration' (2009: 11). This paradigm shift in pedagogy is of course well known in UK Higher Education and the fact that, as Tapscott states, students now 'enjoy a conversation, not a lecture,' seeing themselves as 'collaborators' (2009: 6), is clearly an integral part of many educators' learning strategies at secondary and higher education level. But in the context of an expressly didactic studio training (such as Meyerhold's biomechanics), the argument is clearly more emergent. Indeed, loss of control from the trainer and the levelling out of hierarchies in the studio in many ways undermine the efficacy of such training, compromising rigour and 'depth.'[15] Yet, even in the most vertical of traditions – for instance Chinese Kunju, Keralan Kathakali or Korean Pansori – master-teachers are identifying the quickening of students' expectations and a slow merging of the hitherto clean borders of the digital and the fleshly, Van Dijk's 'integration' of on- and off-line communication.

As Phillip Zarrilli notes in *Psychophysical Acting*, the indigenous practices of South Asia (such as Kathakali) are undergoing significant change. What was once training in a fixed repertoire of physical and dramaturgical conventions, passed on from master to student over several years is now responding to rapid globalization, recognizing that 'young people do not have the time to devote hours to a traditional training' (2009: 81). Konstantinos Thomaidis raises a similar point in relation to Korean vocal practice noting that 'the abundance of relevant online resources' has radically shifted 'the hitherto established microcosm of the teacher-disciple dyad' (Thomaidis 2013: 3). Biomechanics training on the FutureLearn platform may then be viewed simply as another, admittedly more concentrated, example of an international trend: deep training traditions adapting and transforming in conversation with modern technology. The debate is of course much bigger than Keralan, Korean or Russian training in the next part of the 21st century; it extends to the integrity and boundaries of performer training itself. MOOCs are a very small part of this debate, but I have used this form as a case study because it brings into focus several of the purported societal trends we are witnessing now and will experience in concentration in the coming years: the integration of social media behaviours into education; the desire to produce and share (new) cultural forms; the much-needed internationalization and globalization of the Western curriculum; the challenge inclusive learning raises for direct pedagogical hierarchies; the convergence of media and the blurring of everyday and professional life; the desire to study in smaller chunks and the financial necessity to blend online learning with face-face.

In 2009, Tapscott argued current and future students

> prize freedom and freedom of choice. They want to customise things, make them their own. They're natural collaborators, who enjoy a conversation, not a lecture. They'll scrutinise you and your organisation. They insist on integrity. They want to have fun, even at work and at school. Speed is normal. Innovation is part of life.
>
> *(2009: 6–7)*[16]

If 'speed is normal,' then equally important is knowing when and how to slow down, how to resist the quickening of learning as JGR identified above or to break it up and exploit the simultaneities afforded to us by digital media. An acute awareness of time's relationship to learning seems more critical than ever before.

Notes

1 A simple keywords search conducted in January 2014 and once again in November 2017 on YouTube evidences this pattern of growth. In 2014, there were 121,000,000 'How to...' videos, 37,400,000 'Training' videos, 684,000 'Parkour training' videos, 653,000 'Actor training' videos and 3,000 'Meyerhold's biomechanics' videos. In 2017, there were 272,000,000 'How to...' videos, 74,700,000 'Training' videos, 1,140,000 'Parkour training', 2,480,000 'Actor training' videos and 4,280 'Meyerhold's biomechanics' videos.

2 See https://www.mooc-list.com/ for a constantly updated and comprehensive list of MOOCs worldwide, across multiple platforms. See also the paucity of current theatre offerings at: https://www.mooc-list.com/tags/theatre?static=true

3 A two-week version of the longer MOOC called *The Slap: an introduction to Physical Theatre* has run monthly for over a year targeted at Schools, but this does not have live tutor input and interaction.

4 By digital training, I do *not* mean the development of skills and abilities in the use of digital technologies themselves (although that may be a byproduct). Nor am I referring to the vast corpus of training aids designed to develop photo-editing, social media, movie-making, green screen, motion capture or blogging skills. I mean the *appropriation* of digital technologies by a tutor/leader/expert/ambassador/role model to document and/or transmit some level of embodied experience and knowledge.

5 All learner quotations are taken from the comment threads of the three full-length courses run on the FutureLearn platform 2014, 2015, 2018.

6 Conversation with the author on 28 June 2018.

7 As of 2018 on the FutureLearn platform, this flexibility comes at a cost to the learner, who can opt to pay a fee to keep access open to the course materials and for a certificate of participation.

8 LHJ comments:

> I have tried different ways of recording the physical sensations I am feeling while doing the Slap but nothing quite expresses it. Words are inadequate – how do I convey the hot feeling in my head? – the heavy feeling in my feet and hands as they describe arcs through the air? – and then contrast these with the unbelievable lightness of the limbs?– and the bouncy feeling of the pauses with intent? A set of still photos taken by A.N. Other did nothing – video looked clumsy and it didn't feel clumsy – I even tried attaching a video camera to my forehead to see what was seeing. In the end only drawing seemed to capture the sensations.

9 JM comments:

> I took these photos using a continuous shutter – in other words, I performed one continuous, unbroken 'slapping' action while holding the shutter down. The photos – like a classic flipbook – break my holistic action down into the smallest component parts. Look closely, and you will see intention, action and end point clearly represented!

10 111 to be precise, or 3.4%.

11 "The ephochal trend of convergence is the most important trend of the new media in the last 30 to 40 years. It stands for the gradual integration of three types of communication, tele-, data- and mass communication, symbolized by the telephone, the computer, and radio or television respectively" (Van Dijk 2012: 54).

12 See my *Vsevolod Meyerhold* (2018), for an elaboration of Levinsky's training.

13 Conversation with the author on 28 June 2018.

14 Virtual Learning Environments, or VLEs, such as Blackboard, are online repositories of learning resources which allow tutors to release (multimedia) materials to their students incrementally and in tandem with their face-to-face experiences.

15 In his essay 'Keywords for Performer Training,' Simon Murray has recently problematized this term in ways which might be fruitful for this discussion (*TDPT*: 2015): 'For *depth* can we read thickness, consistency, density, girth, width, compactness, opacity, viscosity, consistency, consolidation, intimacy...?'
16 An interesting short critique of Tapscott and his vested interests can be found at: http://www.units.miamioh.edu/psybersite/cyberspace/n-gen/criticism.shtml

References

Cormier, D. (2010) 'What is a MOOC?' YouTube video, found at: https://youtube/eW3gMGqcZQc.

Murray, S. (2015) 'Keywords for performer training,' *Theatre, Dance and Performance Training*, 6(1): 46–58.

Pitches, J. (2014/15/18), *Physical Theatre: Meyerhold's Biomechanics*, MOOC on the FutureLearn Platform, University of Leeds: www.futurelearn.com/courses/physical-theatre.

Pitches, J. (2018), *Vsevolod Meyerhold*, Abingdon: Routledge.

Tapscott, D. (2009) *Grown up Digital: How the Net Generation is Changing the World*, New York: McGraw.

Thomaidis, K. (2013) 'Between Preservation and Renewal: The Use of Recording Devices in Modern *Pansori* Training,' unpublished paper at Performer Training Working Group of TaPRA, Glasgow.

Van Dijk, J. (2012) *The Network Society (3rd ed.)*, London: Sage.

Zarrilli, P. (2009) *Psychophysical Acting: An Intercultural Approach after Stanislavski*, Abingdon: Routledge.

20

FESTIVAL TIME

Kate Craddock

The following discussion derives from embodied and experiential knowledge I have built up over the past decade through immersion in festival culture, both through my role as Founder and Festival Director of GIFT (Gateshead International Festival of Theatre) in North East England, and through experiences and observations at numerous contemporary theatre and performance festivals. Although these festivals themselves are distinctive, and my capacity or role in each has varied (as director, performer, curator, facilitator, adjudicator, participant, audience member, etc.), two characteristics have surfaced as being common to each. First, 'time' in festival contexts is experienced in a complex and disorientating manner; and second, such festivals operate as extraordinarily rich sites for (21st century) performer training. These two assertions are also inextricably linked, as I will go on to propose that it is largely through the way in which time is experienced, that festivals offer an enhanced and visceral 'training' experience. The chapter therefore promotes contemporary theatre festivals as providing a very particular space and time through which to engage in a relevant and long-lasting performer training for the 21st century.

The specific festival experiences cited and drawn on for this chapter, are predominantly small to mid-scale UK and European festivals that either explicitly support and champion experimental, contemporary theatre and performance, and/or offer a platform for emerging artists to showcase or develop their artistic practice. Examples of such festivals, in addition to GIFT, include ACT Festival, Bilbao; BE Festival, Birmingham; OUTNOW! Festival, Bremen; FLARE Festival, Manchester; ITs Festival, Amsterdam, as well as (aspects of) festivals beyond European contexts that operate on significantly larger scales such as Fusebox Festival, Austin and The National Arts Festival in Grahamstown, South Africa.

First though, I open my discussion by highlighting the prevalence of festival culture at this particular moment in time, as well as some of the various common, current understandings of the function and role of festivals. This serves to offer context for the position adopted in this chapter, and to emphasize how this is distinctive from, and offers a contribution to, more readily accepted understandings of the role of festivals. Festival culture is widespread, and the multiple festival experiences on offer across the world, though varied in genre, identity and form, perhaps hold one characteristic in common: they all encourage participants to take 'time out of time' (Falassi 1987: 7). From music festivals designed to deliver hedonism, to street festival parades designed to celebrate specific communities, festivals offer temporary alternative modes of being that are distinctive from everyday life. Indeed, festivals have often been understood in the light of anthropologist Alessandro Falassi's description as 'an event, a social phenomenon, encountered in virtually all human cultures' (1987: 1) and further discussed and theorized as 'a sacred or profane time of celebration' (1987: 2). It is widely accepted that festivals offer a heightened experience, or an alternative to the mundanity of everyday life within a specific culture or community in which they are embedded and from which they grow. They can provide a moment of celebration, encouraging 'communitas' (Turner 1969). They occupy their own space and time, and pertain to their own set of rules, which are distinctive from the 'real world.'

One common critique of festivals that regularly surfaced in conversations and interviews conducted as research for this chapter, was the increased level of commercialization of festival culture, suggesting that festivals have increasingly moved away from being perceived as holding a relationship to something sacred. Rather, 'festival' in the 21st century is more readily viewed as a commodity offered up for consumption by a temporary community of revellers who are ignorant to (or who may wish to buy into) the mass production 'of the experience of freedom' (Toraldo and Islam 2017: 4) that they are being sold. Such observations point to an increasingly cynical and commercial trend in festival culture (largely cited as existing within music festivals, yet there are clear parallels with the commercialization and growth of large-scale theatre festivals such as Scotland's Edinburgh Festival Fringe). Furthermore, another focus of discourse surrounding festivals is the idea of 'Festivalization' coined in the early 1990s by Häusermann and Siebel, to describe the transformative impact that festivals can have on the specific location within which a festival takes place, in particular, whereby the festival is accountable for changing the politics and economics of that area (Zherdev 2014: 6). Such definitions point to a more strategy- or policy-led understanding or function of the role of festival in contemporary society, yet the idea of these festivals offering an alternative to the everyday, or a 'time out of time' remains.

With so many varied understandings of the role of festivals, the environment created and experienced in festival contexts can be interpreted as one that is potentially paradoxical. 'Festival' can be both familiar, in that it is something, as

Falassi highlighted, that is encountered in 'virtually all human culture' (Falassi 1987: 1), yet simultaneously extraordinary, as it is situated outside of everyday lived experience. Additionally, when a (temporary) festival is geographically sited in a location that is seemingly itself unstable, in that it is in a city or area in a process of transition and regeneration (for example GIFT in Gateshead and Fusebox Festival in Austin) then the entire ground on which that (temporary, ephemeral) festival is rooted is also constantly shifting. Time and space in these contexts can therefore be experienced as unfixed, open and confusing. This set of paradoxes, and uncertainties, and the collision of a diverse set of agendas, can serve to enhance the disorientating way in which 'festival time' is experienced and manifests.

In preparation for writing this chapter, I set out to conduct interviews in this array of festival contexts, to talk to other participating artists, programmers and audience members about their own experiencing of time at festivals. Their views and opinions would help to substantiate and challenge my own claims and observations. In order to do this, I made announcements at group discussions and networking events, explaining that I wanted to talk to people about their experience of time; I set up my recording device in bars after shows to capture conversations; I offered to buy people a drink or a coffee in return for their thoughts. However, there was very rarely any time within festival time to really talk about time; not in a way that could substantially and meaningfully feed into this chapter. Rather, as festival participants, we were too busy experiencing the festival; too busy being in the moment to be able to reflect; too late for the next event in the programme; too tired to talk. Those artists, audience members, programmers, festival directors that I did speak to, however, agreed with my initial provocation, that time is experienced at festivals in a way that is complex and confusing. They agreed with my proposition that the all-consuming nature of festivals sets up a strange paradox: on the one hand, festivals are ephemeral, fleeting and take place at a rapid pace; yet on the other, they are so absorbing and all-consuming that they offer the impression and sensation of lasting a much longer period of time than they actually do.

On multiple occasions, I overheard statements that go something along the lines of: 'it's so strange, I feel like I've been here forever,' quickly followed by, 'time has gone so quickly, it is like we only just arrived,' or on departure, 'I know we've only just met, but I feel like I've known you all my life.' Indeed, however ludicrous, I found myself uttering such thoughts. This was 'Festival Time' (Falassi 1987: 4).

> Festival Time imposes itself as an autonomous duration, not so much to be perceived and measured in days or hours, but to be divided internally by what happens within it from its beginning to its end.
>
> *(Falassi 1987: 4)*

Festival Time is largely experienced in two distinct ways. Time is both intensely and carefully structured (through the formality of running to a particular programme of events), but simultaneously, it is very fluid in the ways in which these events are actually experienced.

Indeed, it is very rare that everything runs exactly to plan, something that Fer Montoya, Co- Director of ACT Festival in Bilbao, pointed out in discussion: 'During the festival it is a mess, and the success is that if the things start on time' (Montoya 2015). In fact, it is characteristic of ACT Festival that participants choose to ignore the governing structures in place and rather take ownership, navigating their own way through the festival (by often choosing when to come and go regardless of the programme of events). This looser, more liberating experiencing of time can help to generate an openness among participants, which can in turn instil a sense of belonging, contributing towards creating a community, as will be argued later, can also become a training community.

As Founder and Festival Director of GIFT, this sense of community was something that I specifically set out to cultivate and is something that is often cited as core to participants' experience of the festival.

> The highlight really was the sense of community that the festival engenders in the way it is designed to make it easy for artists and audiences to see lots of work, hang out, and exchange – and the warmth and care with which this is facilitated.
>
> *(Participating Artist, GIFT 2013)*

In order to achieve this and maintain this sense of growing a community year on year, the 'time' at GIFT has become increasingly carefully curated. GIFT operates within a very specific time frame (annually, taking place over three to four days) and within a specific locale (Gateshead). The programme includes performances, workshops and discussions, and a core number of the audience members at all events are made up of the participating artists. Young theatre-makers turn into sponges, soaking up the ideas and strategies played out by more established artists both on stage and off: 'There was a real freedom in participating in the festival, as I was provided with space to make, watch, learn and converse with a number of established artists I had not yet met' (Participating Artist, GIFT 2014). The range of activities on offer, and the subsequent hothouse environment is designed to break down cultural and artistic barriers, encouraging more fluidity between artist and audience. This serves to intensify the complex manner in which both time and training can be experienced and understood.

GIFT participants and audiences might spend their time moving in and out of a five-hour durational performance, into watching a screening of short films, into participating in a workshop, into having a drink with a stranger, only to return back into that same durational performance four hours later where time has seemingly stood still. Each event is programmed with just enough time in between to encourage participants to spend that 'in between' time together. In so doing, they are encouraged to engage in conversations that are charged with the experiences they have just shared, enabling the sought-after temporary festival community to establish. Although this strategy is not made explicit or apparent to participants, this 'in between' time and space for conversation is carefully curated, with 'time for conversations' repeatedly fed back by participating artists as being of significant importance to their experiencing of GIFT.

> I had thrown at me some of the most thought provoking works and IM-PORTANTLY conversations too. I met folk with similar ways of seeing this world and this gave me the ability to envision being a more solid part of this theatre making world, which was inspiring.
>
> *(GIFT participant 2017)*

For GIFT, the particular shaping and experiencing of 'structured time' versus 'in between time' is achieved by creating a programme of festival activity that shifts from formal to informal, from theatre to bar, from gallery to street and from day to night. Festival Time is collapsed, compressed, conflated, and with that, the festival experience can become confusing. There is an intensity to this festival time, which in turn influences how participants choose to exist and behave within this context. Such festival environments premised on community and familiarity, yet also separated from the everyday, can allow participants to occupy an alternative space that is rich with possibility and experimentation. As for GIFT, this can enable an openness in approach that is conducive to taking on new knowledge and new experience. It is in this distinctive 'time out of time' festival offer that participants can become ready for, and open to, 'training,' in whatever guise it comes (Figure 20.1).

It is common practice at GIFT (and many of the festival experiences cited here) that everyone watches everything, moving en mass from one show to the next, deep in conversation or contemplation and making connections. Everyone (mainly) takes part in workshops or discussions during the day, and everyone

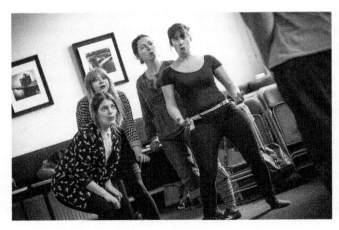

FIGURE 20.1 Voice Workshop, GIFT 2013. Photo: Richard Kenworthy.

eats, drinks and dances together through the night. Remarkably everyone (almost) resurfaces early the next day to start it all over again. This experiencing of festival time was described simply by Fer Montoya, as: '24 hours. 24 hours together' (Montoya 2015). Certainly, there is very little time for sleep. Despite the obvious potential for chaos and general sense of abandon, the impact of this experiencing of time can actually cultivate an environment conducive for meaningful and memorable training to occur, as by operating within the intensity of festival time, a new level of consciousness and awakening take over, and body and mind become ready for anything. Exhausted, but alert and alive.

The training inferred here is not specific to one particular performance style or actor training method. This training does not necessarily offer a deep and enhanced training in one specific approach, or provide expertise in any one field. Instead, the training received through such festivals is far wider reaching, and its legacy can be taken out of the bubble festival world, and into the 'real world.' The training received in these contexts is premised on dialogue and exchange; it awakens curiosity; it teaches how to challenge and question, and to 'keep looking around, not just to look in front' (Participant, Remix Laboratory, National Arts Festival, South Africa). This is a training that is required for the 21st-century contemporary performer, where performers are readily required to be multifaceted practitioners (something that is now understood as common practice particularly in the field of contemporary theatre and performance). Participants are being trained simply through the time that they are spending together and through the proximity and access to each other that the festivals enable.

> Being part of GIFT is really beneficial to my practice, particularly as a young emerging artist. It allows me to network with other artists, often much further ahead in their careers, and attend workshops that allow me to re-evaluate the sort of work I make and why I make it.
>
> *(GIFT participant 2014)*

By encouraging programmed artists at GIFT not only to perform, but also to offer and participate in all the festival activities including workshops, critical feedback discussions, networking opportunities, then the desired festival community is cultivated, operating as a supportive network within which to grow and to train. At GIFT, this festival environment is underpinned by a spirit of generosity, and a commitment to risk-taking and experimentation. As one participating artist at GIFT 2018 commented on the festival: 'the outlook is not one of posturing and being seen, but of generosity, supportiveness and community-building' (Participating Artist, GIFT 2018). Furthermore, for GIFT, this is a diverse community of practitioners, who are at different times in their lives and careers. Established artists and artists of older generations are invited to experience the festival side by side with students, recent graduates and emerging artists. Everyone is operating outside of their perceived familiar context. They are crossing perceived generational, disciplinary and cultural divisions and they are willing to coexist in this shared festival time. Together, they engage in dialogue about the work they are watching, the workshops they are participating in, the food they are sharing and the journeys that have led them here. Being at such different stages and 'time' in their careers is very often what is on participants' minds. Through contact with each other, a festival community is formed, where participants are constantly either looking forward, or reflecting back, whilst simultaneously coming together in the present moment in time within the festival context. Time is no longer straight forward, nor experienced in a linear way.

> During festivals the sense of chronological time disappears into an ever-occurring present ... the past is experienced as return; members participate and recreate a community that feels as if it had always been there.
>
> *(Toraldo and Islam 2017: 4)*

Festivals are bound by time, and notions of time are intrinsic to the very make up of what constitutes a festival. As outlined for GIFT, festivals operate within specific time frames, often appearing on a recurring, cyclical, annual basis. What starts life as a timeline on a spreadsheet will soon become a programme in a festival brochure, and, as the festival itself unfolds, it will become a lived and live experience. Time is mapped out and carefully curated. During the planning stages, significant time is spent considering the impact of how each listing in the programme will sit side by side and how each event will serve to provoke debate, or create a specific post-show atmosphere to further develop a festival community. How festival participants will choose to spend their time and how they will experience time has been mapped out, pre-imagined and timetabled prior to participants' arrival. The construction of festival time enables a sense of community to grow, however, what also lies beneath this construct is a desire to generate an experience that is seemingly free from and distinctive to the routines of everyday time. When this approach succeeds, the usual constructs and constraints of everyday time are abandoned, and a more fluid and powerful Festival Time takes over. This dual, complex and exhausting experiencing of festival time instils a very particular state of being in participants, which invites and enables an opening up to new possibilities and a state conducive to training.

Training, whether intentionally or unintentionally, formal or informal, is what many of these festivals are premised on, and whether articulated as such or not, largely underpins their origins. Certainly, a number of the festivals alluded to here were established for artists at a very particular time in their (emerging) careers. They were specifically for participants who had recently completed their own formal training. Many began life as student theatre festivals, or have grown out of training contexts (with attachments to drama schools and universities), e.g. ACT Festival, Bilbao; ITs festival Amsterdam, with the festival offering a bridge between study and the professional world. As Fer Montoya pointed out in interview:

From the very beginning ACT Festival was born with this aim, especially because it is a festival born and created for people from schools of theatre, and we have a preoccupation, a worry about how to build or help in the professional world the students that finished their studies.

(Montoya 2015)

Where these festivals might differ perhaps in their programming policies, or approach, they are united by their strong desire to launch or sustain careers for artists, often providing young theatre-makers with their first public or professional presentation. As Jacqueline Van Benthem, founder of ITs Festival in Amsterdam and the IYME (International Young Makers Exchange) Network, suggested:

If you go out of the school, it is so important to build up your own international record. How do you do that? I mean it is impossible to do that on your own.

But if you go to all the different festivals, it is so rich; it is an unbelievable opportunity.

(Van Benthem 2015)

Many of these festivals are explicitly designed to be experienced at a very specific time in a young theatre-makers' life, and to fill an important training gap. Unlike festivals whereby 'artists come, do their thing and then go' (Van–Benthem 2015), such festivals depend on the full commitment of the participating artists, who like at GIFT, are invited to attend for the entire duration of the festival, and in so doing, are able to immerse themselves fully in the festival.

Therefore, what is cultivated in festival environments is body and mind in an open state with a readiness and a desire to absorb new experiences. In other words, a desire for training. However, this does not end at the end of the festival. Rather, these new experiences then remain in the memory of participants, ready to unfold in some way in the future. Indeed, training within festival time is played out not only inside the confines of the duration of the festival event, but also beyond. One of the greatest measures of success for festivals is the 'what happens afterwards' and a sense of how the festival experience continues to influence and impact on participants over a longer period of time. For GIFT, many of the experiences and encounters between participants outlive the few days of the festival and instead take on a new life in new collaborations. This is something characteristic also of ACT Festival, Bilbao:

It is typical of the ACT festival that the companies meet each other and work together at some future point of their professional lives.... they offer or present works together for the festival ... there is a company from Belgium who is now working with a company from Andalucía, and they are now making a new project together and this is much bigger than just selling your show because this is related to the creativity process and this is something that transcends the ordinary aims of the ordinary festivals.

(Montoya 2015)

Festivals have a lifespan and impact that can be charted over a far longer period than the few days or weeks that the festival itself plays out. The intensity of the experience ensures there is a legacy and impact that lives on beyond the time frame of the event. Days, weeks, months, years later, and the echoes of the movements encountered in festival workshops and on dance floors, moving collectively with tired feet from one venue to the next, live on in body mind. Images from performances, and of festival faces, of festival routes through an otherwise alien city, reappear in dreams and creative consciousness. New networks and friendships fill social media accounts, entangling participants in a festival web or a collective festival mind. The festival lives on as it infiltrates the return to the 'real world' challenging, and retraining how to now exist in that world (Figure 20.2).

When identifying the key principles that now underpin and govern my practice as a performer, educator and festival director (of listening, participation, cross-cultural communication, resilience and collaboration) and contemplating how and where I was trained in these approaches, I recall very particular times in my life. Notably, the times I spent engaged in festival culture/s. From visiting the Edinburgh Festival as a child; to singing in choral festivals throughout my teens; playing samba in festivals in my early twenties; then performing at Edinburgh Festival Fringe as an emerging theatre-maker; and more recently, participating in multiple European festivals in a range of capacities. The impact of these experiences has been long-lasting, significantly outlasting the few weeks, days or hours spent in any particular festival context. Rather, these have made strong impressions that have informed and trained me over time. They trained me to identify a very specific need and gap in the cultural offer of my own region, and trained me to address that gap: to establish and shape GIFT. This is a varied, non-conventional, yet deeply ingrained training that has emerged over time, and has grown outside a formally structured training time frame. It has been

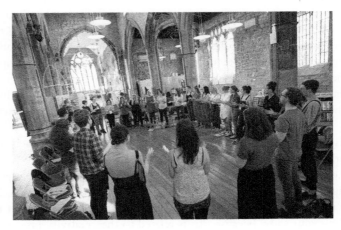

FIGURE 20.2 Great GIFT Welcome, GIFT 2018. Photo: Richard Kenworthy.

a longitudinal training through immersion in festival culture, and remains a lifelong training that continues. It is the diverse and cumulative effect of these experiences that inform my understanding of festivals as extraordinary sites for training, and, by spending more time in these contexts, festivals will undoubtedly continue to train me (and countless others) into the future.

References

Falassi, A. (ed) (1987) *Time out of Time: Essays on the Festival*, Albuquerque, NM: University of New Mexico Press.

Gateshead International Festival of Theatre (GIFT). (2011–2018) Annual festival founded by Kate Craddock, Gateshead, UK.

Montoya, F. (2015) Conversation with Kate Craddock, 4th June.

Toraldo, M.-L. and Islam, G. (2017) 'Festival and organization studies,' *Organization Studies*, 1–14, doi:10.1177/0170840617727785.

Turner, V. (1969) *The Ritual Process: Structure and Anti Structure*, Chicago, IL: Aldine.

Van Benthem, J. (2015) Conversation with Kate Craddock, 5th June.

Zherdev, N. (2014) 'Festivalization as a creative city strategy' [online working paper]. (Doctoral Working Paper Series; DWP14-002). IN3 Working Paper Series. IN3 (UOC). http://journals.uoc.edu/ojs/index.php/in3-working-paper-series/article/view/n14-zherdev/n14-zherdev-en.

21

TIME, FRIENDSHIP AND 'COLLECTIVE INTIMACY'

The point of view of a co-devisor from within Little Bulb Theatre

Eugénie Pastor

I am an artist, theatre-maker and musician. As well as making work on my own, I have been an associate artist at Little Bulb Theatre for the past ten years. Founded in 2008, Little Bulb Theatre is a multi-award-winning company based in the South East of England that tours in the UK and internationally. The company's work intends to 'explore and illuminate minute human details' through performances that 'with humour and sadness will touch, startle and entertain' (*Little Bulb Theatre* 2016). I am a member of the company, but I don't decide on its administrative or artistic direction. I write here from personal and individual experience, simultaneously from outside and from within Little Bulb Theatre. My participation in the company and the relationship I have with each of its members are informed by the length of time we have spent together, as well as by the nature of that time. The blurred delineation between personal, professional and artistic time has proven to be a key condition of the way we developed, consciously or not, a company training. In this provocation, I suggest that our craft was acquired through training informed and shaped by time and friendship, and that this made a 'collective intimacy' possible. I propose that this 'collective intimacy' constitutes one of the particularities of the company's performance style.

As a theatre-maker, I am not formally trained, and neither are any of the artists who compose Little Bulb Theatre. This is the case for several of our contemporaries in the UK. Some of us learnt music, a few studied performance practice and theory at university, but mostly, we learned our craft by doing it. We know how to do what we do because we have spent a lot of time practicing how to do it, and a lot of time doing it. At first, I didn't fully notice I was both co-creating and learning a craft, because along with the rest of the company, I was mostly concerned with finishing and then performing the shows we were making. As time passed, I realized that the skills I was acquiring in Little Bulb Theatre constituted my artistic *training*, which continues to inform the way I make work today and has occasionally been what others have hired me for.

Little Bulb Theatre's performance style is profoundly idiosyncratic: cartoon-like characters, stylized physicality, live music, narrative-led pieces that acknowledge meta-theatricality. I think of this style as 'non-virtuosic': by this I mean it is ambitious and, indeed, virtuosic, but unlike the virtuosity of the trained ballet dancer or guitar player, it is not technically impossible to reproduce. Without professional training, we individually and collectively work at becoming *the best at what we do*. This means mastering scores that we write for ourselves but that are often, at first, too ambitious to be performed by us. This performance style is inevitably connected to the people who make up Little Bulb Theatre. To this day, all Little Bulb Theatre shows have been created, composed and performed by different combinations of the same seven performance-makers (including the company's core of three), under the direction of Alexander Scott, whose influence on the company's style cannot be understated. Another combination of people would have likely generated different outcomes. This is embedded in the company's ethos and approach to theatre-making: Scott elected collaborators for their relationship to one another, not through an audition process, which means we were all brought in because of friendship, not solely for our artistic and professional merits.

I have spent more time working with Little Bulb Theatre than with any other company; in this respect, my training is dependent on the very length of that time spent together. But the fact that friendship is one of the bedrocks of the company suggests that this training didn't solely happen because we spent a long time together: it happened because this time is bound by and constructed through friendship and a specific type of intimacy. It is time spent rehearsing, performing, touring, living, cooking together, celebrating birthdays and weddings, mourning losses, being joyful or grumpy, anxious or carefree, meeting each other's families... The very foundations of the company have depended on material circumstances that, alongside the friendship I have evoked and probably thanks to it, have meant sharing time and space outside of rehearsals and performances, into everyday life. In practice, this has meant that time spent working, and time off, are sometimes not fully demarcated. Many dramaturgical debates, many song arrangements have taken place at the dinner table, on transport to and from venues, when brushing our teeth before bed. In this respect, time spent together, enabled by the comfort and support of our friendship, furthered our training and our practice beyond the rehearsal room. The fact that there is not always a clean-cut delineation between time for work and time for socializing, between private and collective time, has taught me how to be on my own within the collective, how to think beyond myself when I am alone, as well as new forms of intimacy that encompass friendship, siblinghood, professionalism, a support network.[1] I call this 'collective intimacy'.

This 'collective intimacy' permeated the *training* we collectively built and enabled us to acquire a performance and musical style that is as individual and idiosyncratic as it is uniform and collective, for even though similar skills could be acquired, in one way or another, by anybody, there is still a Little Bulb Theatre style that is inherently the company's and the sum of its members' skills, abilities and relationships to one another. This permeates the work and is often commented upon by audience members: our apparent complicity, our evident friendship, blurred the frontier between fact and fiction in *Operation Greenfield*, where it became unclear for several audience members whether or not we were, indeed, the Christian teenagers telling their story in the show, even though the characters were obviously a lot younger than ourselves at the time of impersonating them. This also enabled the emotional undertones of the work to be embraced by some audience members, an intimacy that extended beyond the rehearsal room and the stage and opened up a space to be shared with an audience.

This 'collective intimacy' allows a different form of knowledge, one that extends beyond the distinction between individual and collective, self and other. In his article 'Haptic Geographies: Ethnography, haptic knowledges and sensuous dispositions,' the academic Mark Paterson (2009) suggests that 'the historical emphasis on sight and the optic solidifies perceptual "self"/"other" boundaries between "my" body and others' (781). This, Paterson argues, favours a way of thinking about oneself as 'a cutaneous subject conveniently enveloped … by skin,' something which he argues 'has no neuropsychological basis.' Instead, Paterson says that 'there is no simple inside and outside' because 'the distribution of nerves throughout the body elides any neat distinction between interoception and exteroception in the ongoing nature of somatic experiences' (780). This idea resonates for me because it suggests that there exists a form of knowledge that can be acquired through an understanding of the self that is less impermeable than we think. It asks us to think about what exists within us and between us, as individuals and as members of a group of people collectively responsible for generating new ways of moving, making, performing, being. This shared understanding of the way we move, individually and collectively, is what allows the high levels of ensemble virtuosity and synchronicity in *Orpheus*. Somehow, without actually looking, I know when my co-performers move behind or around me: the scene where I, as Eurydice, chase two of my colleagues holding paper birds, consistently turning to look where they have just left, has now developed in a way where I am able to time my performance with theirs, my movement with theirs. We have collectively developed a high level of control over the scene's comic timing that is, in great part, due to our knowledge of each other's ways of moving.

Acknowledging this suggests that the time I have spent with each member of Little Bulb Theatre and as part of the company has enabled a form of shared embodied knowledge that exists between all of us and as a part of each one of us. This 'collective intimacy' exists when we are together and when we are apart; it is a part of our lives that continues to live with me across geographic and temporal divides. It remains within me, a part of me that is uniquely individual, yet collectively owned.

Note

1 It has also taught us how to effectively draw collective and individual boundaries between these shared aspects of our lives.

References

Little Bulb Theatre (2016) 'Little Bulb Theatre,' www.littlebulbtheatre.com.

Paterson, M. (2009) 'Haptic geographies: ethnography, haptic knowledges and sensuous dispositions,' *Progress in Human Geography*, 33(6): 766–99.

22

TIME MOVES

Temporal experiences in current London-based training for traditional clog and rapper sword dances

Libby Worth

Within the UK and replicated internationally, there are extensive and vibrant networks of amateur dance training practices pursued in leisure time. They exist alongside, and at times interweave with, a broad range of dance and performance training schools/conservatoires with their standardized curricula and established methodologies. One example of such amateur networks, and in microcosm the subject of this chapter, is that of traditional and folk dance. Taking examples of two traditional dances in the UK, the rapper sword dance and clog dancing, originating in North East England coal-mining towns and villages and Lancashire cotton mill towns respectively, the aim of this chapter is to consider how complex experiences of time are infused into every aspect of the trainings. From the hard shoes worn in both dances that ensure their percussive tapping out of time, through the teaching methodology that slows timing to reveal pauses between beats, to the dance performances of under five minutes where time appears to expand to include absurdly complex steps, time is played with, exposed and layered.

The immediacy of temporal experience that surfaces within training is, however, just one of several layers of dancers' relationship to time, since elements existing within the fabric of the dances have endured over a century after their emergence during the industrial revolution in the UK. The rapper and clog dancing that I witnessed/experienced in London are still transmitted to new dancers primarily through direct physical training within team practice, workshops and as I argue, performance. It is tempting to see this as a direct connection through bodily technique to originating communities of the past. Such easy recourse to a simplified version of traditional dance histories would, however, belie the much messier and paradoxical nature of traditional dances and the histories and the accounts that adhere to their current practice. The endurance of dances over time ensures an accumulation of associated stories that could be anecdotal, factual, 'tall,' personal and contradictory. These are not dwelt upon in the following discussion but surface like hauntings, seeping in from the past, equivalent to the manner in which they arise during dance practice/workshops and in the spoken elements of the performances.

There is a paradoxical relationship to time evident in the two London-based examples of traditional dances considered below, which have both manifestly migrated from their originating place, industrial context and time. The dance techniques are imbricated within their history, yet, to successfully perform them, dance respondents assert repeatedly that they need to concentrate fully on the present. Stories from the history of the dances are shaped, selected and enriched with new narratives for contemporary times and specific team's immediate location and character. In engaging through their bodies with past forms, the dancers bring steps and choreographies freshly to contemporary awareness. They are not performing heritage in a rote repetitive fashion, but are caught up, perhaps inevitably, in a spoken and unspoken communication with spectators on ideas, images and feelings triggered by the dynamic currents flowing between past and present within dance performances. In addition, contemporary training in, or transmission of, these dances can give access to principles governing practice that might particularly appeal within the 21st-century cultural terrain that is saturated with artistic drives for celebrity, fame and money. The practice and training for these dances reveal an aesthetic outcome reliant on group rather than individual ownership, together with mutuality and collaboration in the process of contributing to new forms and maintaining earlier choreographies. These traditional dancers' accumulated skill sets, principles and knowledges, which pertain to shared leadership and responsibility for performance quality, have potential application beyond their immediate field of operation. These have clear resonances with professional or amateur dance and theatre ensembles engaged in collaborative performance-making across a variety of genres.

Given that the emphasis for this chapter is on current practices of two traditional dances, the brief historical contexts offered for both of these cannot reflect fully the intricate, multilayered and contested histories typically associated with the study of traditional and folk dances.[1] The two London-based examples of traditional dance training were selected for pragmatic reasons, to allow the kind of regular access to classes, practices and performances that affords time to listen to dance participants and to experience (in the case of the clog dancing only) and observe the dances themselves in some detail. As Judith Hamera makes clear in her study of dance communities in Los Angeles, technique can survive through person-to-person transmissions over long periods of time. Technique 'survives the bodies which enact it, even if the enactments themselves are always and inevitably disappearing. Sometimes technique is an unwanted and burdensome legacy to be resisted; at others it is a generative inheritance' (Hamera 2007: 8). Both dance examples here sit most comfortably within the 'generative inheritance' mode of engagement, having simultaneously strong historical ties whilst continuing to shift and develop, often subtly, in relation to their replacement in time and location from their industrial heritage. Much of the scholarly research into folk and traditional dance practices in England puts emphasis on *place*, with ensuing debates on authenticity, lineages, roots, origins, preservation and ownership. The histories of folk and traditional dances in the UK and their involved relationship to specific communities, sites and regions remain rich territory for scholarship, but in this chapter, the primary perspective is changed from place to time. How do the living traditions of these dances sit within the time continuum of their existence? What surfaces if attention is directed towards time and experience of the temporal in the training of two London-based current practices of traditional dances? There is no question that the speed and precision of clog and rapper dancing demand understanding and memory of rhythms and rhythmic movement patterns of immense complexity and range. How is this experienced in teaching? How is it taught? And what are the kinds of temporal sensibilities called upon and exercised in these practices? Stuart Grant et al., in their introduction to *Performance and Temporalisation: Time Happens*, state that the aim of their text is 'to bring the unique embodied, emplaced, experiential approaches and perspectives which performance allows to the question of the coming-forth of time' (2015: 3). In doing so, they emphasize that 'time is not a given, but is the result of certain processes: of perception, measure, experience and worlding' (3). This is a view that resonates with the approach taken in this chapter which employs a participant and participant-observer methodology to dance training activities to draw on research through doing as well as through description and observation.

It is worth noting from the outset that 'amateur,' as used above, is taken as an encompassing term that denotes activities taking place largely without remuneration or just covering expenses. It implies no reflection of skill level which, as will become obvious, can range from the highest of standards and complexity through to something more basic and quickly learnt. Stephen Knott in a discussion of his text *Amateur Craft: History and Theory* (2015) develops a useful definition:

> The concept amateur, for me, does not represent a person or a group of people (amateurs) but a time-space state, or zone, that we all pass in and out of. It is not defined by poor skill, but by autonomy, or the closest thing to it in the capitalist every day.
>
> *(2016: npn)*

Such a definition is especially appropriate within the context of traditional dance training. It acts as a reminder of how the broader performer training ecology encompassing professional and amateur activities alters, quite dramatically at times, in response to changes in social/cultural fashions, predilections and demands. Which forms become professionalized remain contingent on the values accorded each form and those values are tied closely to political and cultural hierarchies as much as to poplar appreciation. Folk and traditional dance practices were not always relegated to the margins. For instance, the popularity of the music hall and variety theatre during the late 19th century supported traditional dance performers who consequently could earn money teaching others. As these forms of entertainment died out so did that specific economic stream.

Knott's attention to the porosity of amateur/professional practices is helpful in itself as a means of opening up the category of amateur activity and it signals other dualities that come under tension within traditional and folk dance arts. These include differences between work and leisure time – in feeling and motivation, obligation and freedom, play and work, autonomy and control. The types of dances discussed below require regular and rigorous training to achieve the level of performance desired by each group studied. It is not surprising therefore that through history there has been a steady flow between amateur and professional practices within this field as evidenced in early music hall dance, professional teaching of dances and folk dance festival performances. For instance, Ninette de Valois, choreographer, dancer and founder of the Royal Ballet School (RBS) had some experience in, and was aware of, traditional dance practices which she called upon to be included in the RBS curriculum. This element is still taught today at RBS and has usually included both clog dancing and the rapper sword dance.[2]

Both rapper and clog dancing make consistent use of high-intensity rhythmic forms to impact on their audiences. Rhythm is not the same as time, but rhythmic components in performance have the capacity to communicate time states and attitudes. Erica Fischer-Lichte, in writing of the ways in which the 'aesthetic experience in the theatre can be considered a liminal experience' (2007: 231), takes rhythm as a prime example of a structuring device with such transformative potential. She describes rhythm as 'produced by repetition and divergence from that repetition, through beat and break' (231). Given that we all also have internal physiological rhythms about which we may not be aware (unless they falter), Fischer-Lichte suggests that rhythm is 'only able to affect us when we feel it in our bodies, similar to our own bodily rhythms, when we "tune into" them' (231). She suggests that when this happens in performance for an individual, or for many within an audience, it can be a transformative experience. Such impact on spectators is considered in relation to the rapper sword dances only, since the dancers include certain performances (for example monthly 'dance outs' consisting of short dances in different pubs over one evening – 'pub crawls') as an integral part of their training. However, both rapper and clog dance training practices include intense physical dissection of rhythmic structures revealing multiple layers within their experience of time. This can indeed be felt as transformative but equally the disjunctive nature of coexisting 'time-worlds' can surprise and disturb. Both dances' rhythmic structures are imbued with sounds, patterns and materials sourced from their industrial past of the cotton mill and coal mine. The capitalist divide between work and leisure is thus summoned into awareness in the practice rooms of Camden and East London. There is a sense that biological rhythms (both internal patterns and the patterns learnt through music and dance) and structural/organizational rhythms (leisure work) intersect at the level of the body and that it is precisely at this intersection that 'surprises' and 'disturbances' can occur.

Through time

The two dance forms that comprise the primary case-study examples take place in London. Camden Clog are exponents of Pat Tracey's Heel and Toe and other clog dances which were developed by the cotton mill workers of East Lancashire, in North West England. Tracey's repertoire included hornpipes, waltzes and music hall as well as the heel and toe dances, and Camden Clog dance a large selection of all of these (Swift 2018). The group is based in Cecil Sharp House, Camden in North London and comprises at least one dance side (team), dancers who perform/compete individually as well as within the team and regular fortnightly teaching of classes ranging from beginners through intermediate to advanced lessons, as well as day workshops and festival involvement. The second group referenced is Tower Ravens Rapper, who practise in Central London near to the Tower of London, hence their name. They perform rapper sword dances using the traditional short swords that are in fact blunt pliable steel blades with wooden handles at either end, one of which is twistable.[3] Their dances are drawn from the short sword (rapper) practices devised in the coal-mining towns and villages of Northumberland and Durham in the North East of England.

Both the clog and rapper dances emerged from industrial contexts in the 19th and early 20th centuries that were characterized by their tightly controlled and harsh conditions within cramped, loud and often dangerous and unhealthy workplaces. Yet there is evidence in the dances that have come down to us that, despite these long hours, poor pay and dehumanizing conditions, the sounds and materials of industrial life were repurposed as the bases for the stimulation of dance forms and songs. The wooden clogs, for instance, were for common use in the mills to keep feet from the damp floor and wet roads, not originally for dancing. In an industrial setting, time equals money, so clock time in the Lancashire cotton industries regulated the workforces and ensured little room and energy for leisure-time activities. It is perhaps all the more extraordinary that a range of clog-dancing forms should emerge from this environment employing the very materials and resources of the industry itself. The 'Old Lancashire Heel and Toe Clog Dancing,' for example, was developed by cotton weavers who 'took as their footwear the old countryman's clog' resulting in a 'flat-footed style of dancing in which the heel was used as much as the toe to make the sounds' (Camden Clog 2013: back cover). Those sounds were often directly reminiscent of the cacophony of sound made by the cotton mill looms, which of necessity must remain rhythmically perfect. Members of Camden Clog, the first of the dance practices considered here, dance and teach Pat Tracey's Heel and Toe dances from Nelson, East Lancashire, which Tracey learnt as a child, passed down through her family from the mid-19th century (Camden Clog website 2017). The basic steps were learnt by dancers 'who then added their own speciality steps' (Camden Clog 2013: back cover).

Rapper sides were commonly drawn from mining villages and towns of the North East of England, each of which would produce their own variant of the short sword dance. There is a very short silent Pathé News film of one example of these rapper sword dances in practice showing miners emerging directly from the pit at Newbiggin-by-the-Sea, Northumberland (Pathé News Clip 1925). It might have been somewhat staged for the filming but, nevertheless, it evokes the tightness of time for rehearsal and the need to work with sticks as practice short swords (rappers) and in their work clothes to preserve their uniforms and rappers for displays and competitions. Despite the gruelling physical nature of work in the pits, the miners are shown at the end of their shift, flinging down their jackets and moving straight into an energetic routine of dance patterns and jumps whilst linked together with the rapper swords.

The structure and step content of the clog and rapper dancing are very different but they share aspects of significance for the purposes of this chapter. They are strongly percussive, employing hard shoes or clogs (wooden bases with leather uppers) or for the Tower Ravens, military drill shoes with glued on additional soles and heels. Both forms are best performed on wooden flooring or boards. They perform in groups known as sides (although clog dancers do also regularly perform solo) accompanied by traditional folk instruments such as fiddle, whistle or accordion. Tunes for the rapper dances are mainly Irish hornpipes, jigs or waltzes whilst for clog they 'are mostly English folk tunes or popular songs of the time, apart from, for example, the "Lancashire Irish dances"' (also within Tracey's repertoire) (Swift 2018).

The dancers quite often double up to take on the role of musician, so swapping in and out of a side. And, as indicated above, the industrial heritage of both dances is imbued into the forms, rhythms, materials and the stories told about these dances in performance.

Dancing in time

The following accounts expand on notes made from direct experience of learning clog dancing and witnessing rapper sword dancing. The beginners' class at Camden Clog offered the ideal base to start to understand the fast paced and elaborate clog dance performances I had witnessed at festivals, workshops and practices.[4] The beginners' class runs at a slow and steady pace to allow for accuracy in learning foot positioning and rhythm. Unlike many dance forms, the emphasis here is on the aural rather than the visual aesthetic. In discussion with clog dancer and musician Laurel Swift, she said that she had been told 'that in some competitions there would be a 5th judge would sit underneath the stage, to listen to the accuracy of steps rather than watch' (2018). In the contemporary display teams, there is a visual appeal in the costuming and patterning of the group in the performance space but the force and energy comes from the percussive complexity of the clog stepping. To train beginners, the teacher is in the unusual position of having their back to the class. This allows participants to replicate step direction and left/right turn taking most easily. Somewhat unnervingly, as well, I found that the teachers are able to *hear* individual's skill or errors and comment on them without having watched the group. As a beginner, you are given the most basic steps for each dance, along with principles such as 'balancing' on your clogs through having the weight drop forward onto the balls of your feet and making the steps small. The reason for this latter instruction is not immediately obvious but becomes clear on watching a demonstration from the advanced group at the end of each class. There is simply no time to make a large movement with the speed of steps being so intense.

When the new dance to be taught is shown at the start of a set of classes, its speed and intricacy seems impossible to execute and memorize but gradually a new relationship to time develops. It is essential to dance in time with the music being played (slowed down for beginners) and we are taught simple versions of the dances with figures as basic building blocks, which can become progressively more complex as skills improve. Dancing in time seemed to develop another meaning during these classes, especially when watching the advanced groups accurately demonstrating dances of immense intricacy and invention. There was rarely a sound out of place even with musical accompaniment from the accordionist at full speed. The normal beat of clock time seemed to explode open suddenly offering the generous potential for a whole clatter of clog steps to be included in a single moment. I am reminded of one of the teachers at Camden Clog advising me to stop thinking about the steps and to feel the rhythm in the body. She was right. The speed and dexterity required was a holistic experience, even at my very basic level, that required complete attention inside the activity, dancing to time not thinking about the rhythmic structure.

There is a further way that this form of dance appears to operate in time. In my relatively short experience of the beginners' class I have seen participants arrive with no dance background, tap dance or other formal dance training, or a range of other hard shoe forms of traditional dance experience (Welsh clogger, Appalachian dancer, rapper dancers, etc.). In the course of the classes, as the history of the dances unfold during the teaching of steps, participants inevitably become alert to the specifics of this form and how it relates to its industrial heritage. This in itself represents a way in which history (historical experience of time) and personal time (my experience right now of time) can be interwoven in this kind of traditional practice. For example, the distinctive rounded shuffle step[5] of Pat Tracey's style was created originally to help keep the somewhat loose shoes on the feet in fast movements (current clogs are laced and tighter). The clogs were loose to ensure that if a foot was caught in the mill machinery the shoe could be shucked off rather than the foot trapped. The names of many of the steps relate to the sounds of the mill. They are designed to replicate the rhythmic structure and movement of the cotton weaving with taps, shuffles, shunts and a piston-like stamp. To dance these forms is to be in contact, albeit remotely, in both space and time with the drilling of workers to attune their sensibilities to the complex sounds of the mill where any missed beat or irregularity probably signalled a breakdown in the work flow, with direct economic and even disciplinary repercussions. Class participants and tutors with experience of other hard shoe dance forms add to this synchronous awareness through detecting overlapping figures, shared rhythms/music that contribute further to the potentially endless web of references triggered by the dances. Such histories hover in awareness in 21st-century Camden; more prominent, and more obviously enticing for both participants and spectators, is the energy and exhilaration of witnessing something that seems impossible – to insert such varied rhythms and movements through feet on the floor within such a short space of time.

Layered time

The Tower Ravens Rapper similarly pay attention to detail in their dance practices with the aim of producing virtuosic performances but the temporal experience that came through most clearly was of verticality in time. The discussion above, on Camden Clog, considered the linearity of time and how, through practice and skill, intervals of time can be filled with increasingly intricate steps. Despite the minimal use of space, the energy and drama in the rhythmic dynamics have a certain flamboyance. The Tower Ravens Rapper have a similar powerful energy through the percussive downward drive of their shoes on the wooden boards. However, in observing practices and going on a dance crawl around six pubs in Kentish Town, North London, I was most struck by the dense layering of temporalities that became evident during the dancing. These could be termed different 'time-worlds' that coexisted for the duration of the dance revealing how experience exists in vertical as well as linear time. The Australian theatre director and playwright Jenny Kemp has expressed frustration with the societal timeframe she most usually encounters which, as a 'tight linear organization of time amounts to a political act of domination' (1996: 29). Her performances challenge this temporal construction through the creation of a stage space in which multiple time frames are active simultaneously. In so doing, she alerts her audience to the common experience of operating at many levels within a single moment – 'vertical time.' This moves attention away from linear narrative for instance and towards density of awareness with its potential to hold open and active memories, dreams, daily functions and imaginative life all within the same moment. Applied to the rapper dance, this could also include historical memories of the form.

Typically, in a rapper dance pub crawl, there is a group of dancers (eight or so dependent on who is available that night) from which five perform at any one time with a 'Tommy' (a character familiar in most rapper sides along with a 'Betty') and a musician. The Tommy acts variously as introducer, interjector, joker, informer and sixth dancer for a few of the figures. For Tower Ravens Rapper, she wears a Beefeater costume and the musician accompanies the dancers on a fiddle (Figure 22.1).

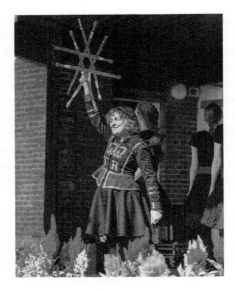

FIGURE 22.1 'Beefeater,' the Tommy for Tower Ravens Rapper. Sidmouth Folk Festival, 2018. Photo: Kyle Baker Photography, courtesy of Tower Ravens Rapper.

The dancers remain linked together with their two handled rapper swords throughout the dance, only opening them to allow the Beefeater in during the final figure. Although the crawl is a series of performances, the dancers explained that these events are seen by them as training. They use these to hone their timing and precision in readiness for the primary competition of the year the Dancing England Rapper Tournament (DERT), which is held annually in a different location each year.

The following contemporaneous description of a small segment of the dance crawl, indicates how temporal awareness can shift from the linear to the vertical within the space of a few minutes. This resonates with Anne Bogart's appreciation of moments of vertical time and how they can be called forth by performance as she describes in the Foreword to this book: 'The experience of vertical time resets and refreshes us' (2019: 4). The accompanying photos show the dance figures particularly well. These were taken of the Tower Ravens performing at Sidmouth Folk Festival, 2018, where they had considerably more light and space.

Tower Ravens Rapper dance crawl 27th July 2017, North London.

It's 22.24 in a very busy pub, The Pineapple in Kentish Town, North London. The punters are sprawled around the narrow areas around the bar that sits centrally in the space. Even just looking for a place to stand as a newly arrived group of 12 or so is tricky.

Relaxed and loudly chatting the pub-goers ooze the feel of downtime, anticipating the next day, Friday, and the start of the weekend. No one is prepared for the next three and half minutes of intensity that is about to explode into their experience.

As a hanger-on and newcomer at such evenings I look anxiously to the organizer wondering where on earth the dance group is going to perform. Unperturbed she surveys the space and points to a corner where a table can be pushed back and a few drinkers moved a little. It still looks tiny and, with the jutting mantle over the fireplace, somewhat hazardous. Undeterred, one of the dance supporters blows a small bugle and in a booming voice announces the name of the Tower Ravens Rapper. The Beefeater takes up the narrative, giving a brief history of the dance and of this all-female side, begun in 2012. The dancers parade into the pub from the street dressed in black and blue symbolizing ravens and, as the fiddler plays, the dance begins in the tiny allotted space (Figure 22.2).

It's fast and furious with feet pounding the beat whilst the swords keep the group linked in their circular chain. The dance, in time with the music, works through a series of figures with the swords operating as the container and aesthetic heart of the dance. Each new figure brings a new element of spectacle to the fore; the jump backwards over the rappers, the turning underneath them in fast flowing patterns, the backward flip of one of the dancers propelled into a high tumble by two others and the final lock where all swords are held triumphantly aloft in the shape of a star (Figure 22.3).

The energy intensifies until the group spins in a fast circle that threatens to spill them into the watching punters. Just the gripping of the rappers controls the centrifugal force (Figure 22.4).

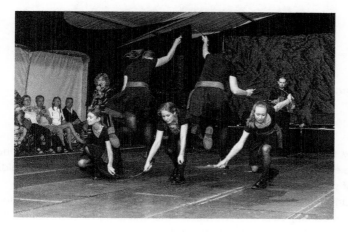

FIGURE 22.2   Tower Ravens jump, Sidmouth Folk Festival. 2018. Photo: Kyle Baker Photography, courtesy of Tower Ravens Rapper.

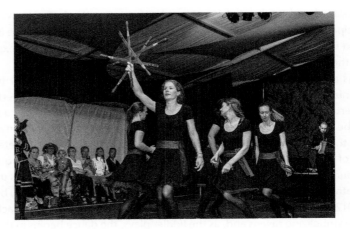

FIGURE 22.3 Tower Ravens with lock, Sidmouth Folk Festival, 2018. Photo: Kyle Baker Photography, courtesy of Tower Ravens Rapper.

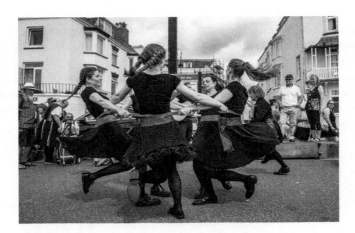

FIGURE 22.4 Tower Ravens spin, Sidmouth Folk Festival, 2018. Photo: Kyle Baker Photography, courtesy of Tower Ravens Rapper.

Finally, the chain is broken for one moment to weave in the Beefeater and the dance ends in a series of twists and turns until she stands forwards holding a star of six locked swords aloft.

During this time, the pub has been in uproar with clapping and shouting of appreciation, calls and whistles at the unfolding of each figure. People stand on chairs to see, take photos and laugh.

This scene was replicated across all six pubs on the crawl, although this final one was the busiest. Even drinkers who looked embarrassed or irritated when they saw costumed dancers enter the pub and prepare, were won over by the skill and intensity of the dancing and the liveliness of the fiddle playing. There is no question that it was an intrusion on their evening but in just those few minutes, I suggest that the dance opened up a layered experience of time. The gentle dynamic of convivial socializing remained, but inserted into this was the much faster and stronger dynamic of the music and dance steps. Multiple references spun into view. Simple actions like shifting around to get a better view or stamping/clapping/cheering to contribute to the atmosphere were combined with taking photos for later, thinking about who to share this with afterwards, talking and gesturing about the event as it happened with friends and absorbing the Beefeater's intermittent commentaries about the rapper sword dancing origins and more recent jokes and stories about this particular dance side.

On this crawl, the dancers were appreciated with vociferous pleasure but each time we entered a new pub I felt nervous. Wasn't it possible that punters would resent an incursion of such a dominant and visceral nature that assaults the senses through visual spectacle, loud sound and vibration of the floorboards? They are not to know for instance, that this encroachment will only last a few minutes before the dancers transform into drinkers just chatting amongst themselves. I wondered how brave the dancers had to feel in order to undertake this and how they would cope if the atmosphere was frosty or even hostile. They are buoyed up, I feel sure, by the pure fun they have in performing and, since they are literally bound together by the swords, no one is over-exposed. If there's an error by one, the collaborative nature of the dance ensures that all must adjust, but with split second timing. However, this method of performing is also supported by the dance's broader cultural history. That is the fearlessness, non-reverential, down-to-earth practicality of the crawl is not specific to Tower Raven Rappers but is a part of very many rapper sides. Typically, these sides perform in festivals/fairs, on the street, in markets, at events to mark specific holidays, at competitions as well as in bars and pubs. They bear with them a non-conformist, disruptive attitude in the sheer high energy, noisy physicality of the dance that seems both spirited, positive and defiant. This forceful, unapologetic approach to entertaining spectators could be seen as an assertion of autonomy in leisure time, as Knott suggested in relation to amateur practices, and freedom from the confines of work time. Tower Ravens Rapper, as an all-female side, operate in a dance terrain that historically was male only and remains male-dominated, although there are now many more female and mixed gender sides. Watching Tower Ravens Rapper delineate their dance space in the crowded pubs (another traditionally male dominated environment) and listening to their stories of participating at DERT, it seemed to me that the confidence gained from 'dancing out' in crawls could be drawn on in a defiant stance if encountering any criticism of women's status in rapper dancing. If this included standing up to resistance to their participation or overly constricting what they could include in their dances, so be it.

The pub-goers, as suggested above, were propelled into an event that had the potential to generate vertical-time experience. In a rather different manner, the dancers too had to deal with complex layering of time within their moments of dance. At a practice session I visited, there happened to be a new participant and it rapidly became clear that the type of teaching I had experienced at Camden Clog was not appropriate for Tower Ravens Rapper. The practice period was precious time for improving the side's technique so that the newcomer, who had some hard shoe clogging experience, was integrated into the dances from the off, being assigned the most straightforward of the roles. The dance was slowed down for her benefit but was used at the same time as a means of reminding more experienced side members of the details of the positioning, placement and travel of both rapper swords and feet. The group works in a collegiate manner with the most experienced members taking it in turns to lead the session and others coming to the fore to offer further detailed critiques (for instance, when I was there, on how to keep the tension in the hands or where to place the gaze) (Figure 22.5).

This sense of shared responsibility is followed through by taking turns in organizing the monthly crawls. It is an approach that suits a dance form that is utterly reliant on each dancer taking charge of their pathway and timing, as any error immediately impacts the whole linked structure. The intensity of focus must be spread therefore between individual actions, group awareness and, when performing, outward gaze to draw in the spectators and to cope with the severely restricted space (Figure 22.6).

The group dance with an element of danger mitigated primarily through intense attention to timing. When talking about their experience of time, dancers in the group mentioned having to have 'strong internal timing and losing outside time' and the need to be 'in exact same time' or 'almost ahead of time, in the next

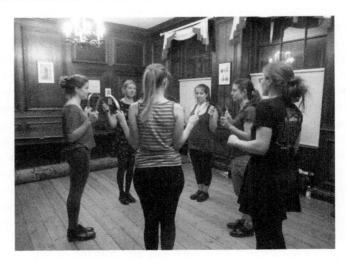

FIGURE 22.5 Tower Ravens Rapper during their practice in Central London, 24 September 2018. Photo: Libby Worth.

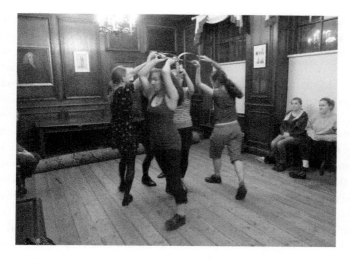

FIGURE 22.6 Tower Ravens Rapper during their practice in Central London, 24 September 2018. Photo: Libby Worth.

moment' (Tower Ravens with Worth 2017). One dancer spoke of not knowing her five moves in one figure, but once in the dance she could do them precisely. These comments resonate with my experience of Camden Clog and indicate that the skill sets cultivated in both contexts could offer useful models within more formal professional training settings, especially in relation to building an ensemble. Ron Smedley notes exactly this valuable impact on the young Royal Ballet School boys to whom he taught rapper dance. Linked together in the rapper was the first time for many of them that they had danced together as opposed to following individually focused training. And, as Smedley wryly noted, this was going to prove essential for many who would end up performing more group dances than solos (Worth 2012: 105–16).

Inclusion of the monthly crawl in the practice programme was (and remains) an essential aspect of training, as it was only through encountering an external reaction that the group could test out their success in maintaining perfect internal timing whilst keeping a partial focus on their surrounds. In embracing vertical time in her performances, Jenny Kemp refers to the need to acknowledge and dialogue with the individual's experience of temporal disjunction. Her focus on activating and making visible inner worlds of dreams and imagination is not replicated in the rapper dances but such resistance to linearity in societal time frame forcefully draws attention to the way that performances have the potential to expose the density of temporal experiences. The Tower Ravens robust interjection of dance into a pub setting could similarly be viewed as a way of disturbing singular experience of time and energetically inserting forceful movement, drama and rhythm in a manner that shatters temporal experience into multiple 'time-worlds' for both performers and spectators.

Both rapper and clog dance training practices are examples of living traditions that can actively replicate dance steps in a contemporary context and innovatively play with historic movement forms. The degree to which they can be said to move away from the 'original' dance choreography and forms varies greatly from one side to another. Tower Ravens Rapper for example, are willing to experiment extensively through being an all-women side bringing new figures and new names for dances/moves arising from their London base. At one event they even completed a rapper dance without their rappers, just imagining their presence. Camden Clog dancers both innovate through individuals/sides recombining and varying Pat Tracey's Heel and Toe routines and they sustain and nurture these dances through teaching. Teaching in itself demands invention and persistence in introducing historic steps to 21st-century dancers with different physicalities and backgrounds who are not steeped in learning through family (in itself another temporal frame) or engrained in the rhythms of mill work. As disciplined leisure-time pursuits, these dances offer an alternative to the strictures of work time whilst generating, through direct physical engagement, new social bonds. There is great potential for the skill sets and principles evident in both the individual and group training for traditional dance forms to interact more fluidly with formal performer training. The impact on performance diversity could replicate that seen develop so impressively in folk music as it encounters and offers reciprocal inspiration to other musical forms, thereby making fresh demands on training. Training for traditional and folk dances is by its very nature a dance with time, which under scrutiny, makes apparent temporal experiences of great diversity and layering.

Acknowledgements

My thanks go to members of Tower Ravens Rapper (especially Hannah and Becky) who have welcomed me to their practices and crawls, and have been willing to answer my many questions. Thanks also to Laurel Swift who has explained many of the details of clog dancing combined with fascinating stories. I am very appreciative of Camden Clog for their inspiring teaching and their dedication to keeping alive such a range of clog dances.

Notes

1 A point that was illustrated substantially in the conference 'The Histories of Morris in Britain' held at Cecil Sharp House, 25–26 March 2017, organized by The Historical Dance Society and The English Folk Dance and Song Society. This link for abstracts and programme also provides an access point to the substantial digital archives of the Vaughn Williams Memorial Library. https://www.vwml.org/events/past-events/special-conferences/3916-the-histories-of-morris-in-britain.

2 See Worth's 'Interviews with Ron Smedley and Simon Rice on the teaching of folk dance and national dances at The Royal Ballet School' and school examples of clog and rapper sword dancing on track 3 DVD (Worth 2012: 105–16).

3 There is no consensus on the origins of the rapper sword. Many believe it to be a tool for scraping the sweat off pit ponies, others think it's a worn down double-handled saw with the remainder of the teeth taken off. Most recently, I heard that it might be a tool used in the pit lift shaft to create a 'rap' sound of the lift descent. If the rhythm was too fast, the descent would then be slowed down.

4 For instance, workshops and displays at Cecil Sharp House, Towersey, Alnwick, Sidmouth Festivals and visits to practices by the Newcastle Kingsmen (Rapper Dances and women's clog dancing), Newcastle Cloggies and Tower Ravens Rapper.

5 This is

as distinct from an ordinary rounded shuffle, which is closer to a tap shuffle. Straight shuffles are where the shuffle goes out and back on the same track, at 12 o'clock, round shuffles are where the shuffle goes out at 2 o'clock and back at 12 o'clock.

(Swift 2018)

The heel-and-toe step itself is rounded.

References

British Pathé. (1925) *Miner Dancers. Newbiggin's Team Straight from Pit's Mouth, Rehearse for Forthcoming National Folk Dancing Display*, Durham, http://www.britishpathe.com/video/miner-dancers-1.

Camden Clog. (2013) *Notation: Pat Tracey's Old Lancs Heel and Toe: Routine A*, London.

———— (2017) Website. http://www.camdenclog.org.uk.

Fischer-Lichte, E. (2007) 'On the threshold. Aesthetic experience in performance,' in Gehm, S., Husemann, P. and von Wilcke, K. (eds) *Knowledge in Motion: Perspectives of Artistic and Scientific Research in Dance*, Bielefeld: transcript Verlag, 227–34.

Grant, S., McNeilly, N. and Veerapen, M. (eds) (2015) *Performance and Temporalisation: Time Happens*, Basingstoke: Palgrave.

Hamera, J. (2007) *Dancing Communities: Performance, Difference and Connection in the Global City*, Basingstoke and New York: Palgrave Macmillan.

Kemp, J. (1996) *Telling Time: Celebrating 10 Years of Women Writing for Performance*, Sydney: Playworks, 29–32.

Knott, S. (2015) *Amateur Craft: History and Theory*, London and New York: Bloomsbury.

———— (2016) 'Presentation notes,' *Amateur Studies Research Forum*, 9th November, Department of Drama, Theatre and Dance, Royal Holloway, University of London.

Swift, L. (2018, 27th September) 'Email exchange with L. Worth,' UK.

Tower Ravens Rapper, website http://towerravens.org.uk/.

Worth, L. (2012) 'Interviews with Ron Smedley and Simon Rice on the teaching of folk dance and national dances at The Royal Ballet School,' in Cave, R.A. and Worth, L. (eds) *Ninette de Valois: Adventurous Traditionalist*, Alton, Hampshire: Dance Books, 105–16.

Worth, L. (2017, 2018) Contemporaneous Notes on Tower Ravens Rapper practices and performances, London and various pubs Kentish Town London: St Michael's Cornhill Church Hall, unpublished.

INDEX

Note: Boldface page numbers refer to tables; italic page numbers refer to figures and page numbers followed by "n" denote endnotes.